The Prediabetes Cookbook and Meal Plan

Easy Low-Sugar, Low-Carb, and Low-GI Recipes to Help Reverse and Manage Diabetes, Including 30-Day and Action Plan

Antonette Batz RD

Copyright © 2024 by Antonette Batz RD

All rights reserved. No part of this publication may be reproduced, distributed, or transmitted in any form or by any means, including photocopying, recording, or other electronic or mechanical methods, without the prior written permission of the publisher, except in the case of brief quotations embodied in critical reviews and certain other non-commercial uses permitted by copyright law. For permission requests, write to the publisher at the address below.

Disclaimer

This book is intended as a general guide to health, wellness, and nutrition. The information contained in this publication is not intended to replace medical advice from a qualified healthcare provider. Always consult your physician or a registered dietitian before making any changes to your diet, exercise, or health plan, especially if you are managing any medical conditions such as prediabetes or diabetes.

While the author and publisher have made every effort to ensure that the information contained in this book is accurate, they assume no responsibility for errors or omissions, nor do they assume liability for any losses, injuries, or damages resulting from the use of this information. The recommendations in this book are based on general guidelines and may not be suitable for all individuals.

Table of Contents

INTRODUCTION 8

CHAPTER 1: PREDIABETES 101 12

    Recognizing the Symptoms and Getting Diagnosed 12

    How Food Affects Blood Sugar: A Simple Guide 13

    The Prediabetic Food Pyramid: What to Eat and What to Avoid 14

    Top 10 Foods to Manage Blood Sugar 15

Chapter 2: The Science Behind Reversing Prediabetes 16

Chapter 3: Breakfast Recipes 20

    Veggie-Packed Egg Muffins 21

    Greek Yogurt Parfait with Chia and Berries 22

    Avocado Toast with Poached Egg 22

    Overnight Oats with Flaxseed and Blueberries 23

    Green Smoothie with Spinach and Almond Butter 23

    Cottage Cheese with Berries and Almonds 24

    Egg White Scramble with Vegetables 24

    Chia Seed Pudding with Almonds and Strawberries 25

    Whole Grain English Muffin with Peanut Butter and Sliced Banana 25

    Sweet Potato and Egg Hash 26

    Omelette with Spinach and Feta 26

    Protein Pancakes with Almond Flour 27

    Quinoa Breakfast Bowl with Berries and Nuts 27

    Smoked Salmon and Avocado Bagel 28

    Low-Carb Egg Muffin Cups 28

Chapter 5: Lunch Recipes 29

Grilled Chicken and Quinoa Salad with Lemon Vinaigrette 29

Turkey and Veggie Wraps with Hummus 30

Mediterranean Lentil Soup with Fresh Herbs 30

Zucchini Noodles with Pesto and Grilled Shrimp 31

FODMAP-Friendly Tuna Salad Lettuce Wraps 31

Chickpea Salad with Tahini Dressing 32

Egg Salad on Whole Grain Crackers 32

Chicken Caesar Salad with Kale 33

Sweet Potato and Black Bean Bowl 33

Quinoa-Stuffed Bell Peppers 34

Salmon Salad with Avocado and Cucumber 34

Spinach and Feta Stuffed Chicken Breast 35

Veggie Stir-Fry with Tofu 35

Cauliflower Rice Bowl with Grilled Chicken 36

Mushroom and Barley Soup 36

Chapter 6: Dinner Recipes 37

Baked Salmon with Roasted Vegetables 37

Turkey Meatballs in Tomato Sauce 38

Stuffed Bell Peppers with Quinoa and Ground Beef 38

Grilled Chicken with Cauliflower Rice 39

Baked Cod with Lemon and Asparagus 39

Vegetable Stir-Fry with Tofu 40

One-Pan Lemon Chicken with Asparagus 40

Beef Stir-Fry with Broccoli 41

Vegetarian Chili with Black Beans and Quinoa 41

Roasted Chicken Thighs with Brussels Sprouts 42

Shrimp and Vegetable Skewers 42

Pork Tenderloin with Roasted Carrots 43

Chickpea and Spinach Curry 43

Tilapia with Sautéed Kale 44

Turkey and Spinach Stuffed Zucchini Boats 44

Chapter 7: Snacks and Sides 45

Roasted Chickpeas with Sea Salt 45

Almond Butter Apple Slices 45

Cucumber and Hummus Bites 46

Greek Yogurt with Walnuts and Cinnamon 46

Low-Carb Veggie Chips with Guacamole 47

Hard-Boiled Eggs with Avocado 47

Carrot Sticks with Almond Dip 48

Edamame with Sea Salt 48

Avocado and Cottage Cheese Bowl 49

Almonds and Dark Chocolate 49

Tuna Salad Lettuce Cups 50

Celery Sticks with Peanut Butter 50

Bell Peppers with Cream Cheese 51

Mixed Nuts and Seeds 51

Tomato and Mozzarella Salad 52

Chapter 8: Desserts and Sweet Treats 53

Low-Sugar Chocolate Avocado Mousse 53

Chia Seed Pudding with Coconut Milk 53

Baked Apples with Cinnamon and Almonds 54

FODMAP-Friendly Almond Flour Cookies 55

Dark Chocolate and Nut Clusters 55

Frozen Yogurt Bark with Berries 56

Peanut Butter Banana Bites 56

Coconut Flour Brownies 57

Ricotta and Berry Parfait 57

Almond Joy Energy Bites 58

Coconut Macaroons 58

Frozen Banana Pops with Dark Chocolate 59

Pumpkin Spice Energy Balls 59

Berry Coconut Smoothie Bowl 60

Cinnamon-Spiced Baked Pears 60

Chapter 9: 30-Minute Meals for Busy Days 61

Stir-Fry with Chicken, Broccoli, and Cashews 61

Sheet Pan Roasted Veggies and Salmon 62

Turkey and Zucchini Skillet 62

Shrimp Tacos with Avocado and Salsa 63

Quick Beef and Vegetable Stir-Fry 63

One-Pan Lemon Garlic Chicken and Green Beans 64

Eggplant Parmesan (Low-Carb) 64

Quick Turkey Lettuce Wraps 65

Vegetable Frittata 65

Tuna Salad with Greek Yogurt 66

Chapter 10: Special Dietary Needs 67

Managing Prediabetes with Food Sensitivities (Gluten-Free, Dairy-Free) 67

Gluten-Free Quinoa and Veggie Stir-Fry 67

Dairy-Free Coconut Chia Pudding 68

Gluten-Free Eggplant Lasagna 68

Dairy-Free Chicken and Veggie Stir-Fry 69

Gluten-Free Oatmeal with Almond Butter 69

Gluten-Free Turkey Lettuce Wraps 70

Dairy-Free Roasted Sweet Potato and Avocado Bowl 70

FODMAP-Friendly Recipes for Sensitive Digestive Systems 71

Low-FODMAP Grilled Chicken Salad 71

FODMAP-Friendly Zucchini Noodles with Pesto 71

Low-FODMAP Carrot and Ginger Soup 72

FODMAP-Friendly Stir-Fried Shrimp 72

Low-FODMAP Baked Salmon with Spinach 73

Low-FODMAP Turkey Meatballs 73

Low-FODMAP Roasted Vegetables 74

Vegetarian and Vegan Options for Prediabetes 74

Vegan Lentil and Quinoa Salad 74

Vegan Stir-Fry with Tofu and Veggies 75

Vegan Sweet Potato and Black Bean Bowl 75

Vegan Chickpea and Spinach Curry 76

Vegan Cauliflower Rice Bowl with Avocado 76

Vegan Black Bean Tacos 77

Vegan Lentil Soup 77

Chapter 11: The 30-Day Action Plan 78

Chapter 12: Bonus 82

30-Day Meal Plan 82

US standard measurement conversion 87

Workout to manage Prediabetes 88

Yoga or Pilates 91

HIIT (High-Intensity Interval Training) 94

Resistance Band Training 96

Conclusion: 99

Final Thoughts and Words of Wisdom from Antonette Batz 100

INTRODUCTION

Imagine taking control of your health and reversing prediabetes—not through restrictive diets or complicated routines, but with simple, delicious meals that nourish your body. This meal will help you change your health one bite at a time, whether you want to manage your blood sugar, lose weight, or feel more energy. This book is full of tasty recipes and useful tips that will show you that eating well doesn't have to be hard and that each meal is a chance to become better.

If your blood sugar levels are higher than usual but not yet high enough to be called type 2 diabetes, you may have prediabetes. It's a very important sign that the body is having trouble handling glucose properly, and if it's not treated, it often leads to full-blown diabetes. The Centers for Disease Control and Prevention (CDC) says that more than one-third of adults in the US have prediabetes. What's even scarier is that most people don't know they have it.

It's hard to tell if someone has prediabetes without a blood test because they don't usually have clear signs. When cells in the body stop responding to insulin, the hormone that helps glucose get into cells, the disease happens. Because of this, glucose levels rise in the blood. While genetic factors play a part, living choices like a bad diet, lack of physical exercise, and extra body weight are major drivers.

The good news is that prediabetes is changeable with lifestyle changes, especially with a healthy diet and regular exercise. Addressing prediabetes early gives the chance to avoid type 2 diabetes and lower the risk of major consequences such as heart disease, stroke, and nerve damage.

Understanding the Importance of Diet in Prediabetes

Diet plays an important part in the control and cure of prediabetes. Your food choices directly affect your blood sugar levels, insulin reaction, and general health. A well-planned meal can help maintain blood glucose levels, improve insulin sensitivity, and lower the chance of getting diabetes.

There are several things that add to the link between food and blood sugar control:

Carbohydrate Intake: Carbohydrates are the main source of energy in your body. However, not all carbs are made equal. Highly processed and refined carbohydrates, such as sugary snacks, white bread, and drinks, can lead to fast spikes in blood sugar. On the other hand, complex carbohydrates like whole grains, veggies, and beans provide a slower, steadier release of glucose, making it easier for your body to control.

Sugar and Insulin: Consuming high amounts of sugar overwhelms the body's insulin reaction, leading to insulin resistance over time. Reducing extra sugars in your diet can help recover normal insulin activity.

Healthy Fats and Protein: Incorporating healthy fats (e.g., avocado, nuts, olive oil) and lean proteins (e.g., chicken, fish, and tofu) into your meals can help balance blood sugar and provide prolonged energy without causing sugar spikes.

Fiber: High-fiber foods slow down the breakdown and uptake of sugar, helping to stabilize blood glucose levels. Fiber-rich foods, such as veggies, fruits, beans, and whole grains, should be a cornerstone of any diet intended to handle prediabetes.

The Role of Low-Sugar, Low-Carb, and Low-GI Foods

When managing prediabetes, a diet high in low-sugar, low-carb, and low-glycemic index (GI) foods can be miraculous. Here's how each of these components plays a role in improving your blood sugar control:

Low-Sugar Foods: Sugar is quickly taken into the body, leading to spikes in glucose and insulin levels. Frequent consumption of sugary foods and drinks increases the chance of insulin resistance, one of the main causes of prediabetes. By minimizing extra sugars and going for natural sweeteners in moderation, you can better control blood glucose and reduce the load on your pancreas.

Low-Carb Foods: Carbohydrates break down into sugar in the bloodstream, so reducing the general amount of carbs in your diet can help avoid blood sugar spikes. A low-carb approach promotes non-starchy veggies, lean meats, and healthy fats, which help to keep blood sugar levels stable and support insulin sensitivity.

Low-GI Foods: The Glycemic Index (GI) tracks how quickly foods raise blood sugar levels. Foods with a low GI cause a slower and more steady rise in blood sugar, while high-GI foods lead to quick jumps. Examples of low-GI foods include most veggies, beans, nuts, and whole grains. Choosing low-GI foods helps to avoid big changes in blood sugar, making it easier to control prediabetes.

How This Book Will Help You Manage and Reverse Prediabetes

This recipe is meant to arm you with the information and tools you need to take control of your prediabetes. Inside, you'll find a collection of delicious, easy-to-prepare meals that focus on low-sugar, low-carb, and low-GI foods. These meals are designed to balance blood sugar, improve insulin sensitivity, and support long-term health goals.

The book also offers complete meal plans suited to different wants and habits, including:

- A 30-Day Meal Plan to kickstart your prediabetes recovery journey.
- A 4-week Action Plan that includes daily meal ideas, tips for controlling hunger, and advice on amount control.
- FODMAP-friendly foods for those with stomach issues.

Whether you're just starting your prediabetes control journey or looking to improve your diet, this book offers expert tips, useful steps, and cooking ideas. Additionally, we'll dive deep into the science behind why certain foods work, giving you confidence in your eating choices. By following the advice in this book, you'll not only learn to handle your prediabetes but also enjoy a variety of healthy and enjoyable meals.

Success Stories: Real People, Real Results

Many people have successfully controlled or even changed their prediabetes by changing their foods and making better living choices.

Here are a few amazing examples:

Sarah's Story: After being diagnosed with prediabetes, Sarah followed a low-sugar, low-carb diet based on the ideas found in this recipe. Over the course of six months, she lost 20 pounds, greatly improved her insulin sensitivity, and was able to bring her blood sugar levels back to the normal range.

Tom's Journey: Tom was at danger of developing type 2 diabetes due to his weight. With the help of the 30-day meal plan in this book, he was able to lower his HbA1c numbers, improve his energy, and even cure his prediabetes diagnosis. Tom thanks his success to the mix of easy, delicious meals and the step-by-step advice offered in this book.

These stories show that with the right method, it is totally possible to recover control of your health and avoid the development of prediabetes.

Tips for Getting the Most Out of This Cookbook

Here are a few methods to maximize the rewards of this cookbook:

Start Small: If you're new to meal planning, begin by adding a few recipes at a time into your weekly routine. Gradually build up to following the meal plans for a full week or month.

Prep Ahead: Planning meals in advance and doing some batch cooking will make it easier to stick to your new eating habits, even when life gets busy. Use the shopping plans given to ease your food trips and ensure you always have healthy items on hand.

Listen to Your Body: Everyone's body acts differently to food. Pay attention to how you feel after meals, and make changes as appropriate. If a particular recipe doesn't work for you, don't be afraid to try another.

Stay Consistent: Managing prediabetes takes a long-term commitment. While it's okay to enjoy rarely, the key to success is regularity. Keep your mind on the bigger picture and use the meal plans as a tool to help your trip.

Track Your Progress: Monitoring your blood sugar levels regularly will help you measure the impact of the changes you've made. Celebrate small wins along the way and change your meal plans as your health improves.

By following the tips and recipes in this book, you'll be well on your way to fixing prediabetes, improving your general health, and having great meals along the way.

CHAPTER 1: PREDIABETES 101

What does prediabetes mean? Causes and Risk Factors

Prediabetes is a metabolic condition where blood sugar levels are increased but not high enough to be labeled as type 2 diabetes. Essentially, it is a warning sign that your body is failing to manage blood glucose effectively, and without help, it may move to full-blown diabetes. Prediabetes is defined by having a HbA1c (a measure of normal blood sugar over the past two to three months) between 5.7% and 6.4%, or a fasting blood sugar reading between 100 and 125 mg/dL.

Causes of Prediabetes are mainly tied to how the body handles glucose. When you eat, the body turns carbs into glucose, a main source of energy. Insulin, a hormone made by the pancreas, lets glucose enter the cells. A condition known as insulin resistance occurs in people with prediabetes, when cells lose their sensitivity to insulin, causing glucose to accumulate in the bloodstream rather than being used for energy. This insulin resistance can stem from different causes:

- **Obesity:** Excess fat, especially around the belly, is highly linked to insulin resistance. Fat cells release inflammatory messages that interfere with the body's ability to use insulin properly.
- **Physical Inactivity:** Regular physical activity helps the muscles use glucose for energy, which lowers blood sugar levels. An idle lifestyle lowers the body's demand for glucose, making it easier for sugar to build in the bloodstream.
- **Genetics:** A family history of diabetes raises the chance of getting prediabetes. Certain racial groups, including African Americans, Hispanics, Native Americans, and Asians, are also at a higher risk.
- **Age:** As people age, their chance of getting prediabetes rises due to changes in body structure, muscle mass, and insulin sensitivity.
- **Diet:** Diets high in processed foods, refined sugars, and sugary drinks can add to the formation of insulin resistance and prediabetes.
- **Hormonal Disorders:** Conditions such as polycystic ovary syndrome (PCOS) and sleep disorders, like sleep apnea, are linked with insulin resistance and can increase the chance of prediabetes.

Recognizing the Symptoms and Getting Diagnosed

One of the difficulties of prediabetes is that it often shows no noticeable signs. Many people with prediabetes are unaware they have it until they undergo regular blood work. However, minor signs that can hint at prediabetes include:

- **Increased Thirst and Frequent urinating:** As blood sugar levels rise, the kidneys work hard to clear extra sugar, leading to more frequent urinating and a subsequent increase in thirst.

- **Fatigue:** With the body fighting to properly utilize glucose for energy, people with prediabetes may feel especially tired or lethargic.
- **Blurred Vision:** Fluctuations in blood sugar levels can cause brief changes in the lenses of the eyes, resulting in blurred vision.
- **Unexplained Weight Loss or Gain:** Some people may experience quick changes in weight without a change in food or physical exercise levels.
- **Slow Healing of Cuts and Infections:** Elevated blood sugar can impair the body's ability to heal cuts effectively.

To identify prediabetes, doctors usually perform the following tests:

- **Fasting Blood Glucose Test:** Blood sugar levels are measured using the fasting blood glucose test after an overnight fast. A fasting blood sugar level of 100–125 mg/dL is indicative of prediabetes.
- **Oral Glucose Tolerance Test (OGTT):** After fasting, patients take a sweet drink, and their blood sugar is monitored at times over the next two hours. Prediabetes is indicated by a blood sugar value between 140 and 199 mg/dL after two hours.
- **Hemoglobin A1c Test:** This test gives an average of your blood sugar levels over the past 2-3 months. An A1c reading between 5.7% and 6.4% signals prediabetes.

How Food Affects Blood Sugar: A Simple Guide

Food plays a crucial role in setting blood sugar levels, especially for people with prediabetes. Here's a simple breakdown of how food changes blood sugar:

Carbohydrates: Carbohydrates are the body's main source of energy and the food most responsible for raising blood sugar. During the process of digestion, carbohydrates are converted to glucose. The more refined or processed the carbohydrate (e.g., white bread, pasta, sugary sweets), the faster it is taken into the bloodstream, leading to spikes in blood sugar levels. Complex carbohydrates (e.g., whole grains, beans, veggies) digest more slowly, giving a steady release of glucose.

Proteins and Fats: These foods do not greatly raise blood sugar levels when eaten alone. Including healthy fats (such as those from avocado, olive oil, and nuts) and lean proteins (such as chicken, fish, and lentils) in meals helps slow down the absorption of carbs, avoiding sharp blood sugar spikes.

Fiber: Foods high in fiber, such as fruits, veggies, and whole grains, help control blood sugar by stopping the processing and uptake of sugar. Soluble fiber, in particular, helps improve insulin reactivity.

Glycemic Index (GI): A ranking system called the Glycemic Index is used to determine how rapidly a meal raises blood sugar levels. Low-GI foods (e.g., leafy greens, beans, nuts) cause a slower, more gradual rise in blood sugar, while high-GI foods (e.g., white bread, candy, potatoes) cause quick spikes. Choosing low-GI foods is an effective way to keep blood sugar levels stable throughout the day.

The Prediabetic Food Pyramid: What to Eat and What to Avoid

The Prediabetic Food Pyramid is a tool to help guide food decisions and amount sizes for people looking to control or cure prediabetes. Unlike the standard food pyramid, which promotes carbs, this form focuses more on veggies, lean meats, and healthy fats.

Base Layer: Non-Starchy Vegetables

What to Eat: Leafy greens (spinach, kale), cruciferous veggies (broccoli, cauliflower), peppers, tomatoes, and cucumbers.

Why: These foods are low in carbohydrates and calories but rich in fiber, vitamins, and minerals that help stabilize blood sugar levels.

Avoid: None — you can eat these easily!

Second Layer: Lean Proteins and Healthy Fats

What to Eat: Chicken, turkey, fish, tofu, beans, eggs, nuts, seeds, olive oil, avocado.

Why: Protein and healthy fats help keep you full and support stable blood sugar levels without causing spikes.

Avoid Saturated and trans fats found in fried foods, fatty cuts of meat, and prepared snacks.

Third Layer: Whole Grains and Low-GI Carbohydrates

What to Eat: Quinoa, brown rice, oats, whole wheat pasta, beans, sweet potatoes.

Why: These are complex carbohydrates that break down slowly in the body, giving a gradual release of glucose and steady energy.

Avoid Refined grains like white bread, cakes, sugary cereals, and normal pasta.

Fourth Layer: Fruits

What to Eat: Berries, apples, pears, citrus fruits (in moderation).

Why: Fruits are a natural source of vitamins, enzymes, and fiber but can still contain a large amount of sugar. Choose low-GI veggies in modest amounts.

Avoid High-sugar foods like bananas, grapes, and dried fruits.

Top Layer: Sweets and Processed Foods

What to Eat: Very sparingly — rare treats in dark chocolate or a small dessert.

Why: These foods can cause quick spikes in blood sugar levels and add to weight gain, which worsens insulin resistance.

Avoid Sugary drinks, candy, baked goods, pop, and other highly processed snacks.

Top 10 Foods to Manage Blood Sugar

Here are the top 10 foods you should add to your diet to help control and cure prediabetes:

- **Leafy Greens:** Rich in fiber, vitamins, and minerals include spinach, kale, and Swiss chard. They are low in calories and carbs, making them an ideal base for any meal.
- **Berries:** Blueberries, strawberries, and raspberries are rich in vitamins and low in sugar compared to other foods, making them great for blood sugar control.
- **Nuts and Seeds:** Almonds, chia seeds, and flaxseeds are full of healthy fats, protein, and fiber, which help control blood sugar levels and keep you feeling full longer.
- **Legumes:** Lentils, chickpeas, and black beans are high in fiber and protein, which help slow down the entry of sugar into the bloodstream.
- **Fatty Fish:** Salmon, mackerel, and sardines are great sources of omega-3 fatty acids, which help lower inflammation and improve insulin sensitivity.
- **Avocados:** This nutrient-dense fruit is rich in heart-healthy fats and fiber, making it a great addition to meals for blood sugar control.
- **Greek Yogurt:** Low in sugar and high in protein, Greek yogurt can be a filling snack that stabilizes blood sugar levels.
- **Whole Grains:** Quinoa, brown rice, and oats are complex carbohydrates that provide long energy without causing a spike in blood sugar.
- **Eggs:** In addition to being strong in protein, eggs also provide vital vitamins and minerals. They are low in carbs and do not affect blood sugar levels.
- **Sweet Potatoes:** Unlike regular potatoes, sweet potatoes are high in fiber and have a lower glycemic index, meaning they won't spike your blood sugar as much.

CHAPTER 2: THE SCIENCE BEHIND REVERSING PREDIABETES

Can You Really Reverse Prediabetes? Understanding the Research

Yes, prediabetes can be restored in many cases, but it takes deliberate lifestyle changes, especially focused on food and physical exercise. Scientific study shows that with the right measures, people with prediabetes can return their blood sugar levels to a normal range, reducing the risk of moving to type 2 diabetes.

The famous Diabetes Prevention Program (DPP) study, supported by the National Institutes of Health (NIH), offers one of the best examples of how lifestyle changes can fix prediabetes. The DPP found that people who followed a healthy diet improved their physical exercise, and achieved moderate weight loss (5-7% of their body weight) cutting their chance of getting diabetes by 58%. This success rate was even higher in older people, hitting a 71% drop for those over 60.

The science behind curing prediabetes is based on improving insulin sensitivity and reducing insulin resistance. Insulin is a hormone that allows cells to receive glucose from the bloodstream. In prediabetes, insulin resistance develops, meaning the body's cells do not respond properly to insulin, causing glucose to build up in the blood. By losing weight, moving regularly, and changing the quality of the food, insulin sensitivity can improve, allowing the body to control blood sugar more effectively. The key is to act early—while prediabetes can be restored if left unchecked, it may grow into type 2 diabetes, a disease that is much harder to cure.

The Role of Low-Glycemic Index (GI) Foods

The glycemic index (GI) is a measure that ranks foods according to how quickly they raise blood sugar levels. The scale runs from 0 to 100, with higher numbers indicating foods that cause a fast spike in blood sugar (high-GI foods) and lower numbers indicating foods that are digested more slowly and cause a steady rise (low-GI foods).

For people with prediabetes, focusing on low-GI foods is important for blood sugar control. These foods help keep a steady flow of glucose into the bloodstream, which lowers insulin spikes and promotes better insulin sensitivity over time. Low-GI foods generally contain more fiber, protein, and good fats, which slow down the digestion process.

Examples of low-GI foods include:

Non-starchy veggies (broccoli, spinach, kale)

Legumes (beans, lentils, chickpeas)

Whole grains (quinoa, barley, oats)

Most fruits (berries, apples, pears)

Dairy items like yogurt and cheese (without extra sugars)

How Low-GI Foods Help Reverse Prediabetes:

- **Stabilizing blood sugar**: Low-GI foods lower fast swings in blood sugar, which are harmful for people with insulin resistance. Stabilizing blood sugar avoids overdoing the body's insulin reaction.
- **Improving insulin sensitivity:** By lowering the need for large amounts of insulin, low-GI foods help prevent insulin resistance from worsening, allowing the body's cells to become more sensitive to insulin over time.
- **Weight control:** Low-GI foods, especially those high in fiber, help with satisfaction and can aid in weight loss, which is a key factor in correcting prediabetes.

Low-Carb vs. Low-Sugar: Which is More Important?

Both low-carb and low-sugar diets can be helpful for controlling prediabetes, but they address blood sugar control in different ways. Let's break down the differences and relative value of each:

Low-Carb Diet:

How it works: A low-carb diet lowers the overall amount of carbs, which are the main source of glucose in the blood. By reducing carbs, you can reduce the spikes in blood sugar that appear after eating.

Benefits: A low-carb diet often leads to better blood sugar control and can promote weight loss. Since prediabetes is linked to insulin resistance, lowering the intake of carbs, especially refined and processed ones, helps lower insulin demand.

Drawbacks: Carbohydrates are not inherently bad. Complex carbs like whole grains, beans, and certain veggies provide important nutrients and fiber, which are helpful for digestion and long-term health. Going too low on carbs may lead to tiredness, and vitamin deficits, and can be difficult to keep long-term.

Low-Sugar Diet:

How it works: A low-sugar diet especially targets foods with added sugars, which are quickly taken by the body and can cause sharp jumps in blood sugar levels. Added sugars are found in many prepared foods, including sugary drinks, sweets, baked goods, and even some savory items like sauces and seasonings.

Benefits: Cutting out extra sugar is one of the fastest and most effective ways to improve blood sugar control. It also drops calorie intake, which can support weight loss. Studies show that increased sugar intake is a major cause of insulin intolerance and metabolic syndrome.

Drawbacks: While removing extra sugars is helpful, naturally occurring sugars in fruits and cheese should not necessarily be avoided unless eaten in excess. These foods also provide important nutrients and are part of a healthy diet.

Which is more important? For correcting prediabetes, a mix of both methods is best. Reducing processed carbohydrates and added sugars will have the most significant effect on lowering blood sugar levels and reducing insulin resistance. A measured approach that limits processed carbs and sugars while adding whole, raw foods is the key to long-term success.

The FODMAP Connection: How It Helps with Gut Health and Blood Sugar

FODMAPs are types of sugars that can be tough for some people to handle. Fermentable oligosaccharides, disaccharides, monosaccharides, and polyols is referred to as FODMAP. These are found in a wide range of foods, including certain fruits, veggies, grains, and dairy products. A low-FODMAP diet is often recommended for people with irritable bowel syndrome (IBS) and other stomach problems.

So, how does the FODMAP link relate to prediabetes and blood sugar control?

Gut health and blood sugar regulation: A recent study shows the link between gut health and metabolic illnesses, including prediabetes. The gut microbiome (the group of bacteria in your food system) plays a key part in regulating blood sugar and insulin sensitivity. A badly working gut, often marked by bloating, gas, and inflammation, can worsen insulin resistance. For people with stomach problems, such as IBS, reducing FODMAPs can improve gut health and, ultimately, improve blood sugar control.

Reducing inflammation: Many people with prediabetes also experience chronic inflammation, which worsens insulin resistance. A low-FODMAP diet may lower gut inflammation, adding to general gains in metabolic health.

Choosing the right FODMAPs: Not all FODMAPs are bad for blood sugar control. Some, like the oligosaccharides found in beans, are rich in fiber and can have a positive effect on blood sugars. The key is to find the FODMAPs that cause stomach pain and handle them while keeping a healthy diet.

While not everyone with prediabetes needs to follow a strict low-FODMAP diet, those with gut issues may benefit from this method as part of a complete plan for improving both stomach and metabolic health.

Building a Sustainable Diet Plan for Long-Term Success

Reversing prediabetes isn't just about short-term changes—it requires building a sustainable, long-term diet plan that you can keep for life. The most effective plan is one that is open, physically balanced, and suited to your individual wants and tastes.

Here's how to make a plan that works for you:

- **Focus on Whole, Unprocessed Foods:** The basis of any good diet plan is to favor whole foods, such as veggies, lean meats, healthy fats, and whole carbs. These foods are generally low in sugar and provide important nutrients that support total health and insulin sensitivity.
- **Incorporate Low-GI and Low-Carb Principles**: While cutting out carbohydrates completely isn't required, focusing on low-GI carbohydrates (like beans, whole grains, and non-starchy veggies) and lowering refined carbs is key. This method helps you keep steady blood sugar levels throughout the day.
- **Limit Added Sugars:** Avoid prepared foods that are high in added sugars. Opt for natural sweeteners like stevia or monk fruit, and enjoy foods in moderation. Reading food labels carefully can help you avoid secret sugars in items like sauces, dressings, and snacks.
- **Balance Macronutrients:** Aim for foods that combine carbs, proteins, and fats. Protein helps stabilize blood sugar, while good fats can improve appetite and insulin sensitivity. Including fiber-rich foods will further slow processing and avoid blood sugar jumps.
- **Meal Prep and Plan Ahead:** Planning your meals in advance is a powerful tool for long-term success. This allows you to control amounts, avoid bad food choices when you're hungry, and ensure you're eating balanced meals that support your goals.
- **Stay Active:** Physical exercise is a key component of controlling prediabetes. Combining regular exercise with a healthy diet improves insulin sensitivity, helps with weight control, and further lowers the chance of diabetes.
- **Be Flexible:** Life is unexpected, and strict diets are hard to keep. The key to long-term success is freedom. If you have an excessive meal, don't feel guilty—just get back on track with your next meal. A healthy living is a race, not a sprint.
- **Monitor Progress:** Regularly check your blood sugar levels, and track your progress. If you notice changes, celebrate them. If things slow, try changing your food or exercise level. Consulting with a healthcare worker or a trained dietitian can help you fine-tune your plan for the best results.

CHAPTER 3: BREAKFAST RECIPES

Why Breakfast is Crucial for Managing Prediabetes

Breakfast is often referred to as the most important meal of the day, and for people controlling prediabetes, this is especially accurate. After a night of fasting, your body needs a healthy lunch to restart your metabolism, manage blood sugar levels, and provide energy for the day ahead. Skipping breakfast or eating the wrong types of foods (such as sugary cereals or sweets) can lead to blood sugar spikes and dips, which can worsen insulin resistance and leave you feeling tired, irritated, and hungry soon after eating.

A well-planned breakfast can help balance blood glucose levels throughout the day, lessen urges, and avoid overeating later on. A healthy breakfast should include low-sugar, high-protein, and high-fiber foods. These nutrients inhibit digestion and the release of glucose into the circulation, avoiding surges and supporting improved insulin sensitivity. By starting your day with nutrient-dense, whole foods, you'll feel more energy, focused, and pleased, which is key to curing prediabetes.

Low-Sugar, High-Protein Options to Kickstart Your Day

When treating prediabetes, breakfast should include a mix of protein, fiber, and healthy fats, with minimal processed carbs and sugars. This helps to slow the flow of glucose into the bloodstream, giving you a steady source of energy. Here are some great low-sugar, high-protein breakfast options:

Veggie-Packed Egg Muffins: These savory muffins are filled with vegetables and protein, making them a full and healthy breakfast. Eggs are high in protein and good fats, while veggies like spinach, bell peppers, and mushrooms provide fiber, vitamins, and minerals. You can make a lot in advance and put them in the fridge for a quick grab-and-go choice.

Greek Yogurt Parfait with Chia and Berries: Greek yogurt is a great source of protein and calcium. By adding chia seeds, which are packed with fiber and healthy omega-3 fats, and antioxidant-rich berries like blueberries or strawberries, you'll make a balanced, low-sugar breakfast that keeps you full until lunch.

Avocado Toast with a Twist: Avocado toast can be a healthy breakfast when made with whole grain bread and paired with a protein source like eggs or smoked salmon. Avocados provide healthy fats and fiber, while whole grains and proteins support normal blood sugar levels.

Green Smoothie with Spinach and Almond Butter: Smoothies can be a handy way to pack in nutrients, but it's important to avoid sugary ingredients. A green shake with spinach, nut butter, and a low-GI fruit like berries or green apples is a great low-sugar, high-fiber pick. Add some protein powder or Greek yogurt to make it more filling.

Overnight Oats with Flaxseed and Blueberries: Overnight oats are a great make-ahead breakfast that is rich in fiber and low in sugar. Oats are a slow-digesting grain, and adding flaxseeds gives healthy omega-3 fats. Blueberries give a natural sweetness while also giving vitamins.

Now, let's dive into the recipes.

These recipes focus on low-sugar, high-protein, and high-fiber ingredients to promote steady blood sugar levels and long-lasting energy. Each recipe is designed to be easy, delicious, and nutrient-dense.

Veggie-Packed Egg Muffins

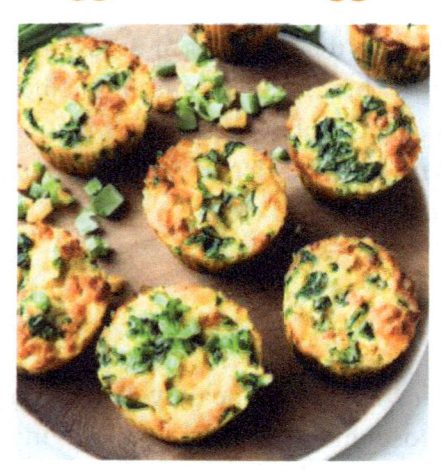

Prep Time: 10 minutes

Cook Time: 20 minutes

Total Time: 30 minutes

Ingredients:

- 6 large eggs
- 1/2 cup spinach, chopped
- 1/2 cup diced bell peppers
- 1/4 cup chopped onions
- 1/4 cup mushrooms, chopped
- 1/4 cup shredded cheese (optional)
- Salt and pepper to taste
- Olive oil spray for greasing

Method:

1. Preheat oven to 350°F (175°C). Grease a muffin tin.
2. Whisk eggs, salt, and pepper in a big bowl.
3. Add spinach, bell peppers, onions, mushrooms, and cheese.
4. Pour mixture into muffin tin.
5. Bake for 15-20 minutes until set and slightly browned.

Nutritional Value (per serving, 1 muffin):

Calories: 90 | Protein: 7g | Carbs: 2g | Fiber: 1g | Fat: 5g

Why It Works: High in protein and fiber, these muffins keep blood sugar steady and can be prepared ahead for busy mornings.

Greek Yogurt Parfait with Chia and Berries

Prep Time: 5 minutes

Total Time: 5 minutes

Ingredients:

- 1 cup plain Greek yogurt
- 1 tbsp chia seeds
- 1/2 cup mixed berries
- 1 tbsp unsweetened shredded coconut (optional)
- 1/4 tsp vanilla extract

Method:

1. Mix chia seeds into Greek yogurt.
2. Top with berries, coconut, and vanilla extract.

Nutritional Value (per serving):

Calories: 200 | Protein: 12g | Carbs: 20g | Fiber: 6g | Fat: 8g

Why It Works: Packed with protein and fiber, this parfait is low in sugar, keeping you full and satisfied.

Avocado Toast with Poached Egg

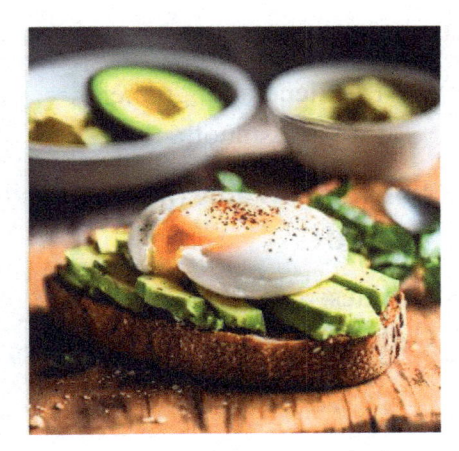

Prep Time: 5 minutes

Cook Time: 5 minutes

Total Time: 10 minutes

Ingredients:

- 1 slice whole grain bread
- 1/2 avocado, mashed
- 1 poached egg
- Lemon juice, salt, and pepper

Method:

1. Toast bread and spread mashed avocado.
2. Top with poached egg, drizzle lemon juice, and sprinkle salt and pepper.

Nutritional Value (per serving):

Calories: 280 | Protein: 10g | Carbs: 24g | Fiber: 8g | Fat: 18g

Why It Works: Healthy fats, fiber, and protein stabilize blood sugar and provide lasting energy.

Overnight Oats with Flaxseed and Blueberries

Prep Time: 5 minutes

Total Time: 5 minutes (plus overnight soak)

Ingredients:

- 1/2 cup rolled oats
- 1 tbsp ground flaxseeds
- 1/2 cup unsweetened almond milk
- 1/2 cup blueberries
- 1/2 tsp cinnamon

Method:

1. Combine oats, flaxseeds, almond milk, and cinnamon in a jar.
2. Stir in blueberries.
3. Refrigerate overnight and enjoy in the morning.

Nutritional Value (per serving):

Calories: 250 | Protein: 8g | Carbs: 40g | Fiber: 10g | Fat: 8g

Why It Works: Oats and flaxseeds provide fiber and protein, ensuring slow digestion and steady blood sugar levels.

Green Smoothie with Spinach and Almond Butter

Prep Time: 5 minutes

Total Time: 5 minutes

Ingredients:

- 1 cup unsweetened almond milk
- 1 cup spinach
- 1 tbsp almond butter
- 1/2 banana
- 1 tbsp chia seeds

Method:

1. Blend all ingredients until smooth.

Nutritional Value (per serving):

Calories: 220 | Protein: 8g | Carbs: 28g | Fiber: 7g | Fat: 12g

Why It Works: Spinach and almond butter provide fiber, protein, and healthy fats for blood sugar control.

Cottage Cheese with Berries and Almonds

Prep Time: 3 minutes

Total Time: 3 minutes

Ingredients:

- 1/2 cup low-fat cottage cheese
- 1/4 cup mixed berries
- 1 tbsp slivered almonds
- A drizzle of honey (optional)

Method:

2. Combine cottage cheese, berries, and almonds in a bowl.
3. Drizzle with honey if desired.

Nutritional Value (per serving):

Calories: 180 | Protein: 15g | Carbs: 10g | Fiber: 2g | Fat: 8g

Why It Works: High-protein cottage cheese and fiber-rich berries make for a filling, low-sugar breakfast.

Egg White Scramble with Vegetables

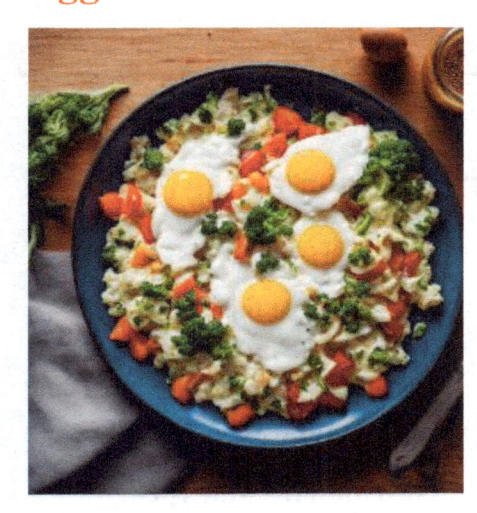

Prep Time: 5 minutes

Cook Time: 5 minutes

Total Time: 10 minutes

Ingredients:

- 4 egg whites
- 1/2 cup chopped spinach
- 1/4 cup diced tomatoes
- 1/4 cup chopped onions
- Olive oil spray

Method:

1. Heat a pan and spray with olive oil.
2. Sauté onions, tomatoes, and spinach until soft.
3. Add egg whites and cook until set.

Nutritional Value (per serving):

Calories: 110 | Protein: 15g | Carbs: 4g | Fiber: 2g | Fat: 3g

Why It Works: Low in calories and carbs, this high-protein scramble keeps blood sugar stable.

Chia Seed Pudding with Almonds and Strawberries

Prep Time: 5 minutes

Total Time: 5 minutes (plus 4 hours to set)

Ingredients:

- 2 tbsp chia seeds
- 1/2 cup unsweetened almond milk
- 1/4 cup sliced strawberries
- 1 tbsp chopped almonds
- 1/2 tsp vanilla extract

Method:

1. In a dish, combine almond milk, vanilla, and chia seeds.
2. Leave it for four hours or all night.
3. Top with strawberries and almonds.

Nutritional Value (per serving):

Calories: 190 | Protein: 6g | Carbs: 16g | Fiber: 10g | Fat: 11g

Why It Works: Chia seeds are rich in fiber and omega-3s, which slow digestion and prevent sugar spikes.

Whole Grain English Muffin with Peanut Butter and Sliced Banana

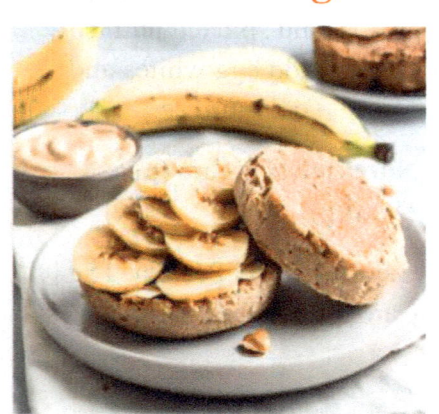

Prep Time: 5 minutes

Total Time: 5 minutes

Ingredients:

- 1 whole grain English muffin
- 1 tbsp natural peanut butter
- 1/2 banana, sliced

Method:

1. Toast the English muffin.
2. Spread peanut butter and top with banana slices.

Nutritional Value (per serving):

Calories: 290 | Protein: 10g | Carbs: 35g | Fiber: 6g | Fat: 12g

Why It Works: Whole grains and peanut butter provide fiber and protein to keep you full and energized.

Sweet Potato and Egg Hash

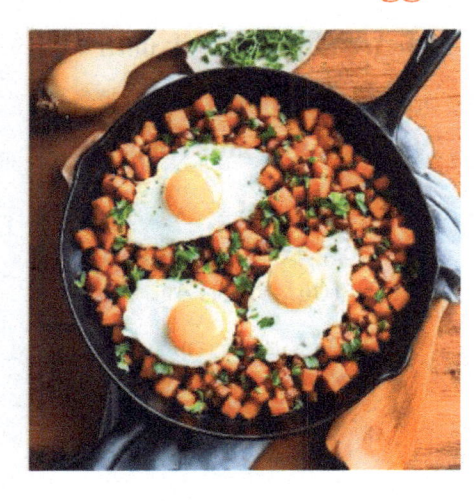

Prep Time: 10 minutes

Cook Time: 15 minutes

Total Time: 25 minutes

Ingredients:

- 1 small sweet potato, diced
- 2 large eggs
- 1/4 cup diced onions
- 1/4 cup diced bell peppers
- Olive oil spray

Method:

1. Heat a pan and cook sweet potato, onions, and bell peppers until soft.
2. Crack eggs over the potatoes and cook until set.

Nutritional Value (per serving):

Calories: 250 | Protein: 12g | Carbs: 35g | Fiber: 6g | Fat: 8g

Why It Works: Sweet potatoes are a low-GI carb, paired with eggs for protein and fiber.

Omelette with Spinach and Feta

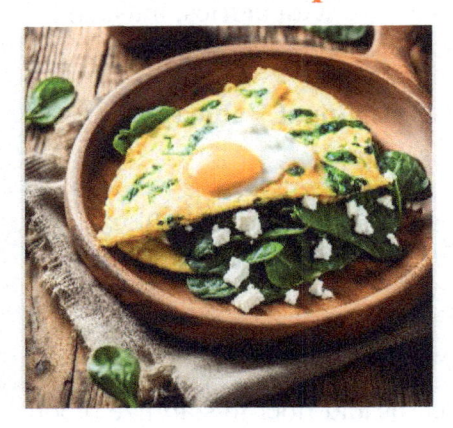

Prep Time: 5 minutes

Cook Time: 5 minutes

Total Time: 10 minutes

Ingredients:

- 2 large eggs
- 1/4 cup spinach
- 2 tbsp crumbled feta cheese
- Salt and pepper to taste

Method:

1. Whisk the eggs and add a pinch of salt and pepper.
2. Pour into a heated pan and add spinach and feta.
3. Fold omelet and cook until eggs are set.

Nutritional Value (per serving):

Calories: 200 | Protein: 14g | Carbs: 3g | Fiber: 1g | Fat: 14g

Why It Works: High in protein and healthy fats, this omelet supports stable blood sugar.

Protein Pancakes with Almond Flour

Prep Time: 5 minutes

Cook Time: 5 minutes

Total Time: 10 minutes

Ingredients:

- 1/2 cup almond flour
- 1/4 cup protein powder
- 1/4 tsp baking powder
- 1 large egg
- 1/4 cup unsweetened almond milk

Method:

1. Mix all ingredients to form a batter.
2. Pour batter into a heated pan and cook until bubbles form.
3. Flip and cook until golden brown.

Nutritional Value (per serving):

Calories: 250 | Protein: 18g | Carbs: 10g | Fiber: 4g | Fat: 18g

Why It Works: Almond flour and protein powder keep carbs low and protein high for blood sugar control.

Quinoa Breakfast Bowl with Berries and Nuts

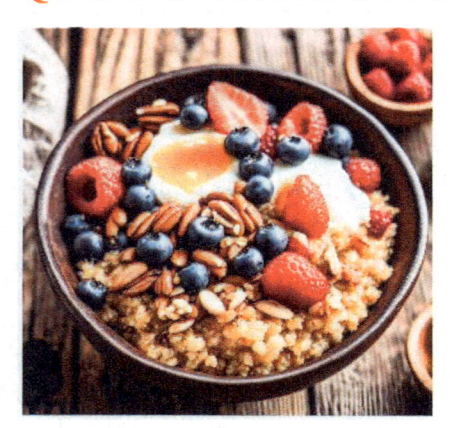

Prep Time: 5 minutes

Cook Time: 15 minutes

Total Time: 20 minutes

Ingredients:

- 1/2 cup cooked quinoa
- 1/4 cup mixed berries
- 1 tbsp chopped nuts
- 1 tsp honey

Method:

- Combine cooked quinoa with berries, nuts, and honey.

Nutritional Value (per serving):

Calories: 220 | Protein: 6g | Carbs: 35g | Fiber: 5g | Fat: 8g

Why It Works: Quinoa is a protein-rich grain that provides complex carbs and fiber to stabilize blood sugar.

Smoked Salmon and Avocado Bagel

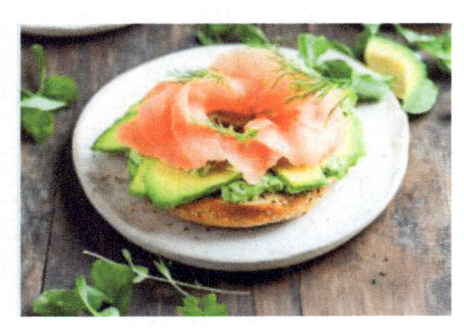

Ingredients:

- 1 whole grain bagel thin
- 2 oz smoked salmon
- 1/4 avocado, sliced
- A squeeze of lemon juice

Method:

1. Spread avocado on the toasted bagel.
2. Garnish with smoked salmon and a splash of lemon juice.

Nutritional Value (per serving):

Calories: 250 | Protein: 14g | Carbs: 28g | Fiber: 6g | Fat: 10g

Prep Time: 5 minutes
Total Time: 5 minutes

Why It Works: Smoked salmon provides healthy fats and protein, while the bagel adds fiber.

Low-Carb Egg Muffin Cups

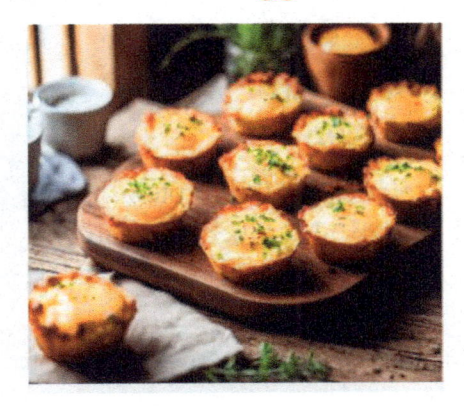

Total Time: 30 minutes

Ingredients:

- 6 eggs
- 1/4 cup chopped spinach
- 1/4 cup diced ham
- 1/4 cup shredded cheese
- Salt and pepper

Method:

1. Preheat oven to 350°F.
2. Whisk eggs with salt and pepper.
3. Add spinach, ham, and cheese.
4. Transfer the mixture into a muffin tin and bake for twenty minutes.

Nutritional Value (per serving):

Calories: 150 | Protein: 12g | Carbs: 1g | Fiber: 1g | Fat: 10g

Prep Time: 10 minutes
Cook Time: 20 minutes

Why It Works: These low-carb muffins are high in protein and perfect for managing blood sugar.

CHAPTER 5: LUNCH RECIPES

These lunch recipes are created with low-sugar, high-protein, high-fiber, and complex carbohydrate ingredients to promote stable blood sugar levels and long-lasting energy. They are simple to prepare, nutritious, and delicious.

Grilled Chicken and Quinoa Salad with Lemon Vinaigrette

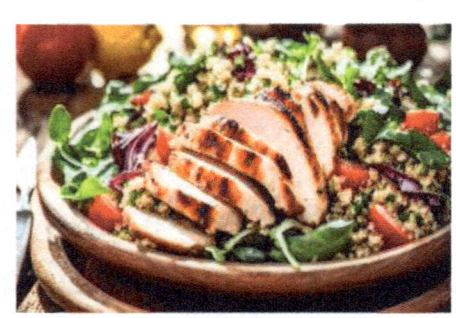

Prep Time: 10 minutes

Cook Time: 20 minutes

Total Time: 30 minutes

Ingredients:

- 1 cup cooked quinoa
- 4 oz grilled chicken breast
- 1/4 cup chopped cucumber
- 1/4 cup cherry tomatoes, halved
- 2 tbsp crumbled feta cheese
- 2 tbsp olive oil
- 1 tbsp lemon juice
- Salt and pepper to taste

Method:

1. In a large bowl, combine cooked quinoa, grilled chicken, cucumber, cherry tomatoes, and feta.
2. Whisk together olive oil, lemon juice, salt, and pepper to make the vinaigrette.
3. Drizzle the vinaigrette over the salad and toss gently to mix everything together.

Nutritional Value (per serving):

Calories: 350 | Protein: 25g | Carbs: 30g | Fiber: 6g | Fat: 14g

Why It Works: Quinoa is a complex carb rich in protein and fiber, which helps keep blood sugar stable, while lean chicken provides satisfying protein.

Turkey and Veggie Wraps with Hummus

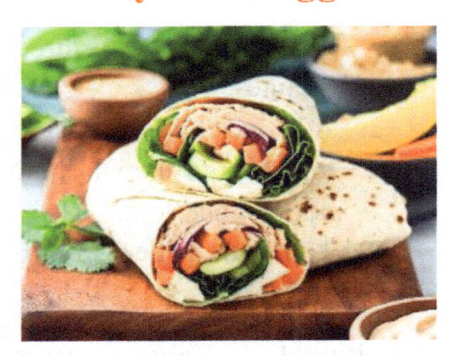

Prep Time: 5 minutes

Total Time: 5 minutes

Ingredients:

- 1 whole wheat tortilla
- 4 oz sliced turkey breast
- 2 tbsp hummus
- 1/4 cup sliced bell peppers
- 1/4 cup shredded carrots
- 1 handful spinach leaves

Method:

1. Spread hummus on the whole wheat tortilla.
2. Layer with turkey, bell peppers, carrots, and spinach.
3. Roll the tortilla tightly and cut it in half.

Nutritional Value (per serving):

Calories: 300 | Protein: 22g | Carbs: 32g | Fiber: 7g | Fat: 10g

Why It Works: The whole wheat wrap provides complex carbs, while turkey and hummus offer protein and fiber, preventing sugar spikes.

Mediterranean Lentil Soup with Fresh Herbs

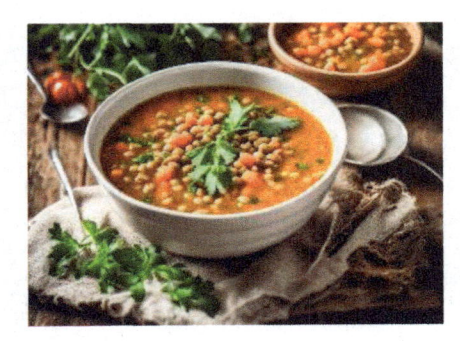

Prep Time: 10 minutes

Cook Time: 25 minutes

Total Time: 35 minutes

Ingredients:

- 1 cup dried lentils
- 4 cups vegetable broth
- 1/2 cup diced tomatoes
- 1/4 cup diced onions
- 2 cloves garlic, minced
- 1 tsp cumin
- 1 tsp olive oil
- Fresh parsley for garnish

Method:

1. Cook the onions and garlic in olive oil until they become soft and fragrant.
2. Add lentils, vegetable broth, tomatoes, and cumin.
3. Let it simmer for twenty-five minutes, or until the lentils are tender.
4. Garnish with fresh parsley and serve.

Nutritional Value (per serving):

Calories: 280 | Protein: 18g | Carbs: 40g | Fiber: 15g | Fat: 4g

Why It Works: Lentils are high in fiber and protein, which helps slow the absorption of carbs and promotes stable blood sugar levels.

Zucchini Noodles with Pesto and Grilled Shrimp

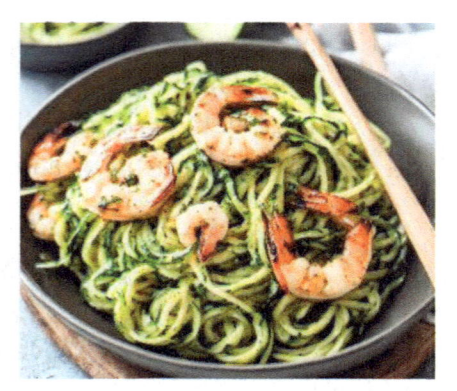

Prep Time: 10 minutes

Cook Time: 10 minutes

Total Time: 20 minutes

Ingredients:

- 2 medium zucchinis, spiralized
- 6 large shrimp, grilled
- 2 tbsp pesto (store-bought or homemade)
- 1 tbsp olive oil
- 1/4 cup cherry tomatoes, halved

Method:

1. Warm olive oil in a pan and sauté the zucchini noodles for two to three minutes.
2. Add pesto and cherry tomatoes to the zucchini noodles and toss.
3. Top with grilled shrimp and serve.

Nutritional Value (per serving):

Calories: 300 | Protein: 25g | Carbs: 10g | Fiber: 4g | Fat: 18g

Why It Works: Zucchini noodles are a low-carb alternative to pasta, while shrimp provides lean protein. The beneficial fats in the pesto aid in regulating blood sugar levels.

FODMAP-Friendly Tuna Salad Lettuce Wraps

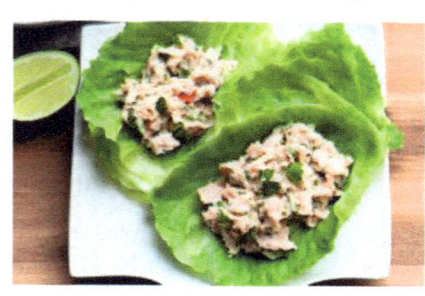

Prep Time: 5 minutes

Total Time: 5 minutes

Ingredients:

- 1 can tuna in water, drained
- 2 tbsp Greek yogurt
- 1 tbsp Dijon mustard
- 1/4 cup diced cucumber
- 1 tbsp chopped chives
- 2 large lettuce leaves

Method:

1. Mix tuna, Greek yogurt, mustard, cucumber, and chives in a bowl.
2. Place the tuna salad in the lettuce leaves and wrap them up.

Nutritional Value (per serving):

Calories: 180 | Protein: 22g | Carbs: 3g | Fiber: 1g | Fat: 8g

Why It Works: Tuna is rich in protein and omega-3 fats, while lettuce wraps keep the dish low-carb and light, helping to manage blood sugar.

Chickpea Salad with Tahini Dressing

Prep Time: 10 minutes

Total Time: 10 minutes

Ingredients:

- 1 cup canned chickpeas, rinsed
- 1/2 cup diced cucumbers
- 1/2 cup cherry tomatoes
- 2 tbsp tahini
- 1 tbsp lemon juice
- 1 tsp olive oil
- Fresh parsley for garnish

Method:

1. In a bowl, combine chickpeas, cucumbers, and tomatoes.
2. Whisk together tahini, lemon juice, olive oil, and parsley to make the dressing.
3. Mix the salad with the dressing and serve.

Nutritional Value (per serving):

Calories: 280 | Protein: 10g | Carbs: 34g | Fiber: 10g | Fat: 14g

Why It Works: Chickpeas are a great source of fiber and plant-based protein, helping to control blood sugar levels while keeping you full.

Egg Salad on Whole Grain Crackers

Prep Time: 5 minutes

Cook Time: 10 minutes (boiling eggs)

Total Time: 15 minutes

Ingredients:

- 2 hard-boiled eggs, chopped
- 1 tbsp Greek yogurt
- 1 tbsp Dijon mustard
- 1 tbsp chopped celery
- Whole grain crackers for serving

Method:

1. Mix chopped eggs, Greek yogurt, mustard, and celery in a bowl.
2. Serve egg salad on whole grain crackers.

Nutritional Value (per serving):

Calories: 250 | Protein: 12g | Carbs: 20g | Fiber: 4g | Fat: 15g

Why It Works: Eggs are a complete protein source, and the whole grain crackers add fiber, ensuring a balanced, low-sugar lunch.

Chicken Caesar Salad with Kale

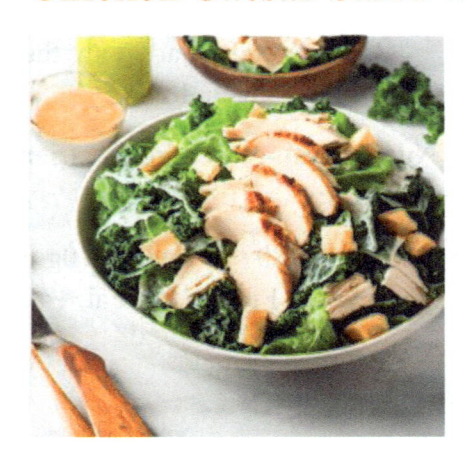

Prep Time: 10 minutes

Cook Time: 10 minutes (grilling chicken)

Total Time: 20 minutes

Ingredients:

- 4 oz grilled chicken breast
- 2 cups chopped kale
- 2 tbsp Caesar dressing (light or homemade)
- 1 tbsp grated Parmesan cheese
- 1/4 cup croutons (optional)

Method:

1. Toss chopped kale with Caesar dressing.
2. Top with grilled chicken, Parmesan, and croutons.

Nutritional Value (per serving):

Calories: 320 | Protein: 30g | Carbs: 10g | Fiber: 3g | Fat: 18g

Why It Works: Kale provides fiber and essential nutrients, while grilled chicken adds protein. A lighter Caesar dressing helps keep the salad lower in calories and sugar.

Sweet Potato and Black Bean Bowl

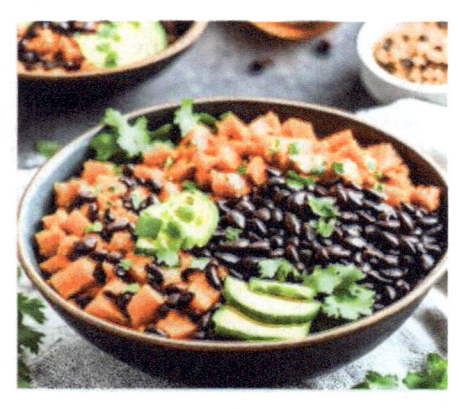

Prep Time: 10 minutes

Cook Time: 20 minutes

Total Time: 30 minutes

Ingredients:

- 1 small sweet potato, diced
- 1/2 cup black beans
- 1/4 cup diced avocado
- 2 tbsp salsa
- 1 tsp olive oil

Method:

- Roast diced sweet potato in olive oil at 400°F (200°C) for 20 minutes.
- In a bowl, combine roasted sweet potatoes, black beans, avocado, and salsa.

Nutritional Value (per serving):

Calories: 350 | Protein: 10g | Carbs: 50g | Fiber: 14g | Fat: 12g

Why It Works: Sweet potatoes and black beans are high in fiber and complex carbohydrates, which help maintain stable blood sugar levels.

Quinoa-Stuffed Bell Peppers

Prep Time: 10 minutes

Cook Time: 25 minutes

Total Time: 35 minutes

Ingredients:

- 2 large bell peppers, halved and deseeded
- 1/2 cup cooked quinoa
- 1/4 cup black beans
- 1/4 cup diced tomatoes
- 2 tbsp shredded cheese (optional)
- 1 tsp olive oil

Method:

1. Preheat oven to 375°F (190°C).
2. Mix cooked quinoa, black beans, and tomatoes.
3. Stuff bell peppers with the mixture, top with cheese, and bake for 25 minutes.

Nutritional Value (per serving):

Calories: 290 | Protein: 12g | Carbs: 45g | Fiber: 12g | Fat: 8g

Why It Works: Quinoa and black beans provide complex carbs and protein, while bell peppers add fiber and vitamins.

Salmon Salad with Avocado and Cucumber

Prep Time: 10 minutes

Total Time: 10 minutes

Ingredients:

- 4 oz cooked salmon
- 1/2 avocado, sliced
- 1/4 cup diced cucumber
- 1 tbsp olive oil
- 1 tbsp lemon juice
- Salt and pepper

Method:

1. Combine salmon, avocado, and cucumber in a bowl.
2. Sprinkle with salt and pepper and drizzle with lemon juice and olive oil.

Nutritional Value (per serving):

Calories: 350 | Protein: 25g | Carbs: 8g | Fiber: 6g | Fat: 24g

Why It Works: Salmon is high in protein and omega-3 fats, which support heart health and help manage blood sugar levels.

Frozen Yogurt Bark with Berries

Prep Time: 5 minutes

Total Time: 5 minutes (plus 2 hours freezing time)

Ingredients:

- 1 cup plain Greek yogurt
- 1 tbsp honey (optional)
- 1/4 cup mixed berries (blueberries, strawberries)
- 1 tbsp chia seeds

Method:

1. Spread Greek yogurt evenly on a parchment-lined baking sheet.
2. Top with berries, chia seeds, and a drizzle of honey.
3. Freeze for two hours or until firm, then break into pieces.

Nutritional Value (per serving):

Calories: 120 | Protein: 10g | Carbs: 12g | Fiber: 3g | Fat: 3g

Why It Works: Greek yogurt is high in protein, while berries add natural sweetness and antioxidants. Chia seeds provide fiber and omega-3s to keep blood sugar steady.

Peanut Butter Banana Bites

Prep Time: 5 minutes

Total Time: 5 minutes

Ingredients:

- 1 medium banana, sliced
- 2 tbsp natural peanut butter
- 1/4 tsp cinnamon

Method:

1. Spread peanut butter on banana slices and sprinkle with cinnamon.
2. Stack the slices to make mini sandwiches, or enjoy as-is.

Nutritional Value (per serving):

Calories: 190 | Protein: 5g | Carbs: 25g | Fiber: 4g | Fat: 10g

Why It Works: Bananas provide fiber and natural sweetness, while peanut butter offers healthy fats and protein to slow sugar absorption.

Coconut Flour Brownies

Prep Time: 10 minutes

Cook Time: 20 minutes

Total Time: 30 minutes

Ingredients:

- 1/4 cup coconut flour
- 2 tbsp unsweetened cocoa powder
- 1/4 cup melted coconut oil
- 1/4 cup monk fruit sweetener or preferred low-calorie sweetener
- 3 eggs
- 1/2 tsp vanilla extract
- 1/4 tsp baking soda

Method:

1. Preheat oven to 350°F (175°C).
2. Mix coconut flour, cocoa powder, coconut oil, sweetener, eggs, vanilla, and baking soda in a bowl.
3. Pour batter into a greased baking dish and bake for 20 minutes.

Nutritional Value (per serving, 1 brownie):

Calories: 150 | Protein: 4g | Carbs: 8g | Fiber: 4g | Fat: 12g

Why It Works: Coconut flour is low-carb and high in fiber, making these brownies a great option for blood sugar control while still enjoying a rich, chocolaty treat.

Ricotta and Berry Parfait

Prep Time: 5 minutes

Total Time: 5 minutes

Ingredients:

- 1/2 cup ricotta cheese (low-fat)
- 1/4 cup mixed berries (blueberries, raspberries)
- 1/2 tsp vanilla extract
- 1 tsp honey (optional)

Method:

1. Layer ricotta cheese with mixed berries and drizzle with honey.
2. Add vanilla extract for extra flavor.

Nutritional Value (per serving):

Calories: 180 | Protein: 8g | Carbs: 16g | Fiber: 4g | Fat: 8g

Why It Works: Ricotta is high in protein and low in carbs, while berries provide fiber and natural sweetness to make this parfait a healthy, blood sugar-friendly dessert.

Almond Joy Energy Bites

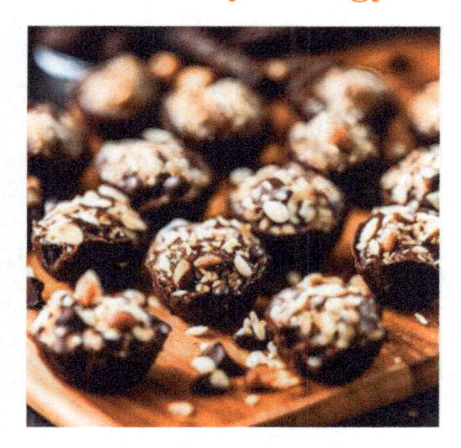

Prep Time: 10 minutes

Total Time: 10 minutes

Ingredients:

- 1/2 cup almond flour
- 2 tbsp unsweetened shredded coconut
- 1 tbsp almond butter
- 1 tbsp cocoa powder
- 1 tbsp maple syrup (optional)
- 1 tsp vanilla extract

Method:

1. In a bowl, mix all ingredients until well blended.
2. Roll into small balls and refrigerate for 10 minutes to set.

Nutritional Value (per serving, 2 bites):

Calories: 120 | Protein: 4g | Carbs: 8g | Fiber: 3g | Fat: 10g

Why It Works: These energy bites are packed with healthy fats, fiber, and protein, making them a satisfying treat without causing blood sugar spikes.

Coconut Macaroons

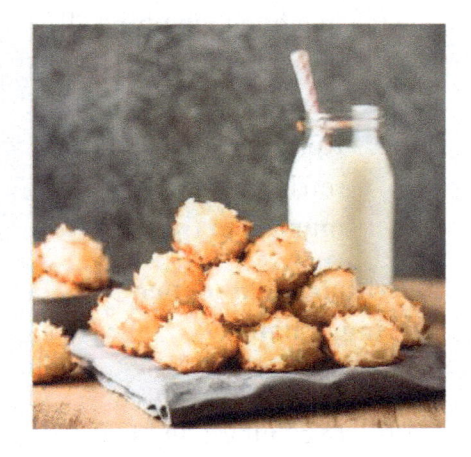

Prep Time: 10 minutes

Cook Time: 15 minutes

Total Time: 25 minutes

Ingredients:

- 2 cups unsweetened shredded coconut
- 2 egg whites
- 1/4 cup monk fruit sweetener (or your preferred low-calorie sweetener)
- 1 tsp vanilla extract
- 1/4 tsp salt

Method:

1. Preheat oven to 325°F (165°C).
2. Beat egg whites with salt until frothy. Stir in shredded coconut, sweetener, and vanilla.
3. Shape into little mounds and transfer to a baking sheet covered with paper.
4. Bake for 12-15 minutes until golden brown.

Nutritional Value (per serving, 2 macaroons):

Calories: 120 | Protein: 3g | Carbs: 5g | Fiber: 4g | Fat: 10g

Why It Works: Coconut is naturally low in carbs and rich in fiber and healthy fats, which support blood sugar control. These macaroons provide a sweet treat without the sugar spike.

Frozen Banana Pops with Dark Chocolate

Prep Time: 5 minutes

Cook Time: 5 minutes (melting chocolate)

Total Time: 10 minutes (plus freezing time)

Ingredients:

- 1 banana, cut into thirds
- 2 oz dark chocolate (70% cocoa or higher), melted
- 1 tbsp chopped almonds or walnuts

Method:

1. Put a wooden stick into every slice of banana.
2. Dip the bananas into the melted dark chocolate and sprinkle with chopped nuts.
3. Put on a tray covered with parchment paper and freeze for two hours.

Nutritional Value (per serving, 1 pop):

Calories: 140 | Protein: 2g | Carbs: 20g | Fiber: 4g | Fat: 8g

Why It Works: Bananas offer natural sweetness and fiber, while dark chocolate and nuts add healthy fats and antioxidants, making this a satisfying dessert that won't spike blood sugar.

Pumpkin Spice Energy Balls

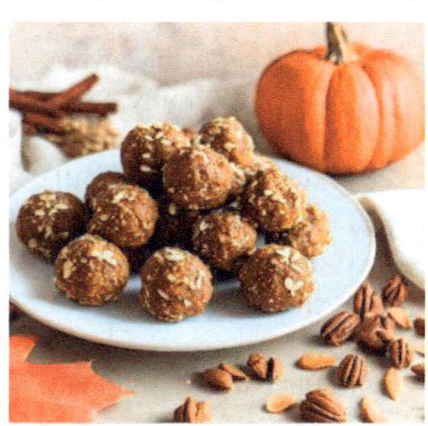

Ingredients:

- 1/2 cup rolled oats
- 1/4 cup pumpkin puree (unsweetened)
- 2 tbsp almond butter
- 1 tbsp chia seeds
- 1 tbsp maple syrup (optional)
- 1/2 tsp pumpkin spice

Method:

1. In a bowl, combine all the ingredients and well mix.
2. Roll into small balls and refrigerate for 10 minutes to firm up.

Nutritional Value (per serving, 2 balls):

Calories: 140 | Protein: 4g | Carbs: 18g | Fiber: 4g | Fat: 6g

Prep Time: 10 minutes

Total Time: 10 minutes

Why It Works: Pumpkin is low in carbs and packed with fiber, while oats and chia seeds provide complex carbs and healthy fats. This dessert is filling and helps keep blood sugar steady.

Berry Coconut Smoothie Bowl

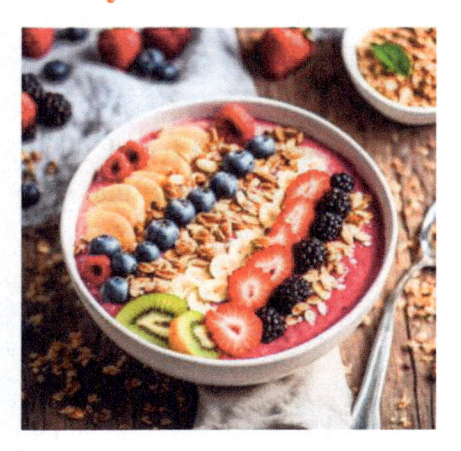

Prep Time: 5 minutes

Total Time: 5 minutes

Ingredients:

- 1/2 cup frozen mixed berries
- 1/4 cup unsweetened coconut milk
- 1/2 cup Greek yogurt
- 1 tbsp chia seeds
- 1 tbsp unsweetened shredded coconut

Method:

1. Blend frozen berries, coconut milk, and Greek yogurt until smooth.
2. Transfer into a dish and garnish with shredded coconut and chia seeds.

Nutritional Value (per serving):

Calories: 200 | Protein: 10g | Carbs: 25g | Fiber: 7g | Fat: 8g

Why It Works: This smoothie bowl combines antioxidant-rich berries with Greek yogurt for protein and chia seeds for fiber. It's naturally sweet without added sugar and helps control blood sugar levels.

Cinnamon-Spiced Baked Pears

Prep Time: 5 minutes

Cook Time: 20 minutes

Total Time: 25 minutes

Ingredients:

- 2 medium pears, halved and cored
- 1 tsp cinnamon
- 1 tbsp chopped walnuts
- 1 tsp honey (optional)

Method:

1. Preheat oven to 350°F (175°C).
2. Place pear halves in a baking dish and sprinkle with cinnamon, walnuts, and honey.
3. Bake for 20 minutes until pears are soft and golden.

Nutritional Value (per serving, 1 pear half):

Calories: 100 | Protein: 1g | Carbs: 22g | Fiber: 4g | Fat: 3g

Why It Works: Pears are naturally sweet and high in fiber, making them a perfect dessert for managing blood sugar. Walnuts add healthy fats, while cinnamon may help regulate blood sugar.

CHAPTER 9: 30-MINUTE MEALS FOR BUSY DAYS

Easy and Quick Recipes to Make When You're Short for Time

These recipes are perfect for busy days when you need something quick, healthy, and blood sugar-friendly. They can all be prepared in 30 minutes or less, using simple, wholesome ingredients that keep you full and energized.

Stir-Fry with Chicken, Broccoli, and Cashews

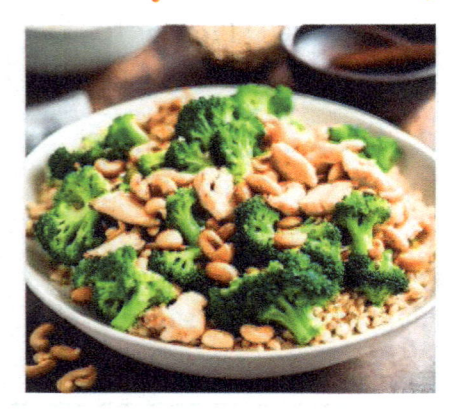

Prep Time: 10 minutes

Cook Time: 15 minutes

Total Time: 25 minutes

Ingredients:

- 1 chicken breast, thinly sliced
- 1 cup broccoli florets
- 1/4 cup cashews
- 1 tbsp olive oil
- 1 tbsp low-sodium soy sauce
- 1 clove garlic, minced
- 1/2 tsp ginger (optional)

Method:

1. Heat olive oil in a pan and sauté chicken for 5 minutes.
2. Add garlic, broccoli, and soy sauce, stir-frying for another 5-7 minutes.
3. Stir in cashews and cook for an additional 2 minutes.
4. Serve hot.

Nutritional Value (per serving):

Calories: 320 | Protein: 28g | Carbs: 10g | Fiber: 3g | Fat: 18g

Why It Works: Chicken provides lean protein, and the broccoli adds fiber, helping to stabilize blood sugar. Cashews add healthy fats for satiety and flavor.

Sheet Pan Roasted Veggies and Salmon

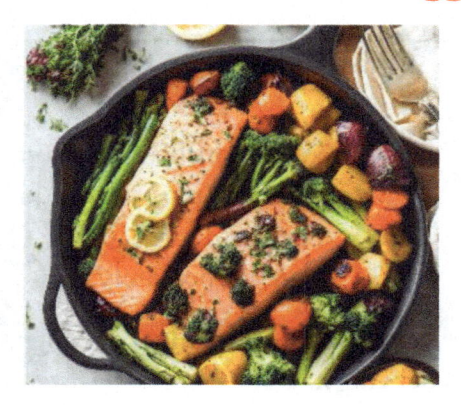

Prep Time: 10 minutes

Cook Time: 20 minutes

Total Time: 30 minutes

Ingredients:

- 1 salmon fillet (4 oz)
- 1/2 cup Brussels sprouts, halved
- 1/2 cup diced sweet potato
- 1 tbsp olive oil
- 1 tsp rosemary
- Salt and pepper to taste

Method:

1. Preheat oven to 400°F (200°C). On a baking sheet, arrange the fish and veggies.
2. Season with salt, pepper, rosemary, and olive oil.
3. Roast for 20 minutes, until the salmon flakes easily with a fork and vegetables are tender.

Nutritional Value (per serving):

Calories: 350 | Protein: 30g | Carbs: 25g | Fiber: 6g | Fat: 18g

Why It Works: Salmon is a great source of omega-3 fatty acids and protein, while the sweet potatoes and Brussels sprouts provide fiber and complex carbohydrates to maintain blood sugar balance.

Turkey and Zucchini Skillet

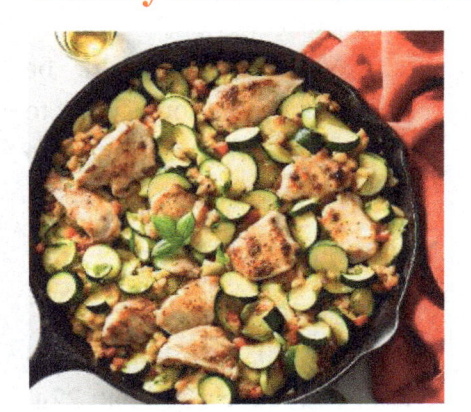

Prep Time: 5 minutes

Cook Time: 20 minutes

Total Time: 25 minutes

Ingredients:

- 8 oz ground turkey
- 1 zucchini, diced
- 1/4 cup diced onions
- 1/4 cup diced bell peppers
- 1 tbsp olive oil
- 1 tsp Italian seasoning
- Salt and pepper to taste

Method:

1. Heat olive oil in a skillet and cook onions, bell peppers, and zucchini until soft.
2. Add ground turkey, season with Italian seasoning, salt, and pepper.
3. Cook for eight to ten minutes, or until turkey is browned.

Nutritional Value (per serving):

Calories: 320 | Protein: 26g | Carbs: 10g | Fiber: 3g | Fat: 18g

Why It Works: Ground turkey is a lean source of protein, and the vegetables are low in carbs but rich in fiber, making this dish a perfect quick, low-sugar meal.

Shrimp Tacos with Avocado and Salsa

Prep Time: 10 minutes

Cook Time: 10 minutes

Total Time: 20 minutes

Ingredients:

- 6 large shrimp, peeled and deveined
- 2 small whole wheat tortillas
- 1/2 avocado, sliced
- 1/4 cup salsa
- 1 tbsp olive oil
- 1/2 tsp cumin

Method:

1. Heat olive oil in a pan and cook shrimp with cumin for 3-4 minutes per side.
2. Warm tortillas and top with shrimp, avocado slices, and salsa.
3. Serve immediately.

Nutritional Value (per serving):

Calories: 300 | Protein: 20g | Carbs: 28g | Fiber: 6g | Fat: 14g

Why It Works: Shrimp is a lean protein source, and avocado provides heart-healthy fats. The whole wheat tortillas offer fiber to keep blood sugar levels steady.

Quick Beef and Vegetable Stir-Fry

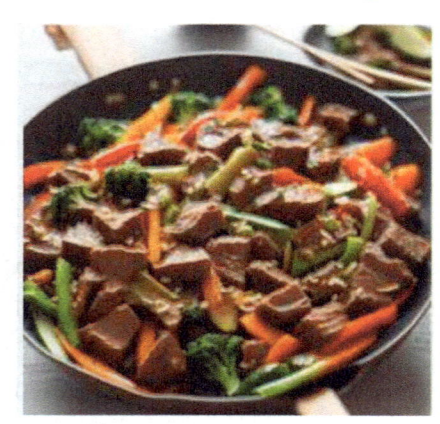

Prep Time: 10 minutes

Cook Time: 10 minutes

Total Time: 20 minutes

Ingredients:

- 4 oz lean beef strips
- 1/2 cup broccoli florets
- 1/4 cup sliced bell peppers
- 1 tbsp sesame oil
- 1 tbsp low-sodium soy sauce
- 1 tsp garlic, minced

Method:

1. In a pan over medium heat, sauté the meat strips until browned.
2. Add broccoli, bell peppers, garlic, and soy sauce.
3. Vegetables should be stir-fried for five to seven minutes in order to soften them.

Nutritional Value (per serving):

Calories: 350 | Protein: 28g | Carbs: 10g | Fiber: 3g | Fat: 22g

Why It Works: Lean beef provides high-quality protein, while the fiber-rich vegetables help keep you full and support stable blood sugar levels.

One-Pan Lemon Garlic Chicken and Green Beans

Prep Time: 10 minutes

Cook Time: 20 minutes

Total Time: 30 minutes

Ingredients:

- 1 chicken breast, thinly sliced
- 1 cup green beans
- 1 tbsp olive oil
- 2 cloves garlic, minced
- 1 tbsp lemon juice
- Salt and pepper to taste

Method:

1. Heat olive oil in a pan and cook chicken slices until browned, about 6-8 minutes.
2. Add garlic and green beans, cooking for an additional 5 minutes.
3. After adding a little lemon juice and seasoning with salt and pepper, serve.

Nutritional Value (per serving):

Calories: 280 | Protein: 30g | Carbs: 6g | Fiber: 3g | Fat: 14g

Why It Works: This dish is rich in lean protein and low in carbohydrates, perfect for keeping blood sugar stable. Green beans are high in fiber and vital elements.

Eggplant Parmesan (Low-Carb)

Prep Time: 10 minutes

Cook Time: 20 minutes

Total Time: 30 minutes

Ingredients:

- 1 medium eggplant, sliced
- 1/2 cup marinara sauce (no sugar added)
- 1/4 cup shredded mozzarella cheese
- 2 tbsp olive oil
- 1 tsp Italian seasoning

Method:

1. Preheat oven to 400°F (200°C). Brush eggplant slices with olive oil and sprinkle with Italian seasoning.
2. Roast eggplant for 10 minutes.
3. Top with marinara sauce and mozzarella, and bake for another 10 minutes until cheese is melted.

Nutritional Value (per serving):

Calories: 250 | Protein: 10g | Carbs: 10g | Fiber: 4g | Fat: 18g

Why It Works: Eggplant is low in carbohydrates and high in fiber. The dish offers a satisfying, low-carb alternative to traditional pasta dishes while keeping your blood sugar in check.

Quick Turkey Lettuce Wraps

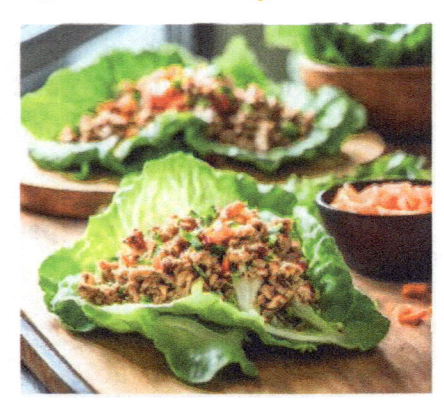

Prep Time: 5 minutes

Cook Time: 10 minutes

Total Time: 15 minutes

Ingredients:

- 6 oz ground turkey
- 2 large lettuce leaves
- 1/4 cup diced bell peppers
- 1/4 cup shredded carrots
- 1 tbsp soy sauce (low sodium)
- 1 tbsp olive oil

Method:

1. In a skillet with heated olive oil, sauté ground turkey for eight minutes.
2. Add bell peppers, carrots, and soy sauce, cooking for an additional 2 minutes.
3. Spoon turkey mixture into lettuce leaves and serve as wraps.

Nutritional Value (per serving):

Calories: 260 | Protein: 25g | Carbs: 10g | Fiber: 3g | Fat: 14g

Why It Works: These low-carb lettuce wraps provide lean protein and fiber from the vegetables, making them a quick and blood sugar-friendly meal.

Vegetable Frittata

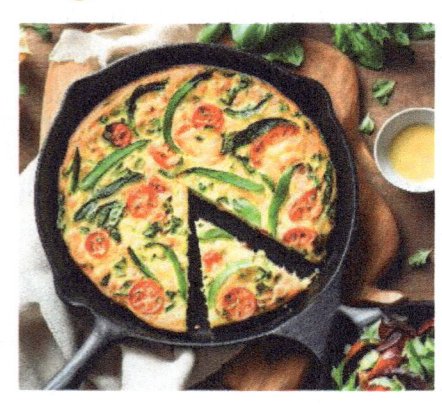

Prep Time: 5 minutes

Cook Time: 20 minutes

Total Time: 25 minutes

Ingredients:

- 4 large eggs
- 1/4 cup diced zucchini
- 1/4 cup diced tomatoes
- 1/4 cup diced onions
- 1 tbsp olive oil
- 1/4 tsp black pepper

Method:

1. Preheat oven to 350°F (175°C). Heat olive oil in a skillet and sauté onions, zucchini, and tomatoes for 5 minutes.
2. Beat eggs with pepper and pour over vegetables.
3. Bake in the oven for 15 minutes until eggs are set.

Nutritional Value (per serving):

Calories: 220 | Protein: 14g | Carbs: 8g | Fiber: 2g | Fat: 16g

Why It Works: Eggs are a high-protein, low-carb option that's perfect for stabilizing blood sugar. The added vegetables increase the fiber content, promoting fullness and better blood sugar control.

13	Quinoa Breakfast Bowl with Berries and Nuts (p. 27)	Veggie Stir-Fry with Tofu (p. 35)	Chickpea and Spinach Curry (p. 43)	Bell Peppers with Cream Cheese (p. 51)	Pumpkin Spice Energy Balls (p. 59)
14	Smoked Salmon and Avocado Bagel (p. 28)	Cauliflower Rice Bowl with Grilled Chicken (p. 36)	Tilapia with Sautéed Kale (p. 44)	Mixed Nuts and Seeds (p. 51)	Berry Coconut Smoothie Bowl (p. 60)
15	Low-Carb Egg Muffin Cups (p. 28)	Mushroom and Barley Soup (p. 36)	Turkey and Spinach Stuffed Zucchini Boats (p. 44)	Tomato and Mozzarella Salad (p. 52)	Cinnamon-Spiced Baked Pears (p. 60)
16	Greek Yogurt Parfait with Chia and Berries (p. 22)	Grilled Chicken and Quinoa Salad with Lemon Vinaigrette (p. 29)	Baked Salmon with Roasted Vegetables (p. 37)	Roasted Chickpeas with Sea Salt (p. 45)	Low-Sugar Chocolate Avocado Mousse (p. 53)
17	Avocado Toast with Poached Egg (p. 22)	Turkey and Veggie Wraps with Hummus (p. 30)	Turkey Meatballs in Tomato Sauce (p. 38)	Almond Butter Apple Slices (p. 45)	Chia Seed Pudding with Coconut Milk (p. 53)
18	Overnight Oats with Flaxseed and Blueberries (p. 23)	Mediterranean Lentil Soup with Fresh Herbs (p. 30)	Stuffed Bell Peppers with Quinoa and Ground Beef (p. 38)	Cucumber and Hummus Bites (p. 46)	Baked Apples with Cinnamon and Almonds (p. 54)
19	Green Smoothie with Spinach and Almond Butter (p. 23)	Zucchini Noodles with Pesto and Grilled Shrimp (p. 31)	Grilled Chicken with Cauliflower Rice (p. 39)	Greek Yogurt with Walnuts and Cinnamon (p. 46)	FODMAP-Friendly Almond Flour Cookies (p. 55)

20	Cottage Cheese with Berries and Almonds (p. 24)	FODMAP-Friendly Tuna Salad Lettuce Wraps (p. 31)	Baked Cod with Lemon and Asparagus (p. 39)	Low-Carb Veggie Chips with Guacamole (p. 47)	Dark Chocolate and Nut Clusters (p. 55)
21	Egg White Scramble with Vegetables (p. 24)	Chickpea Salad with Tahini Dressing (p. 32)	Vegetable Stir-Fry with Tofu (p. 40)	Hard-Boiled Eggs with Avocado (p. 47)	Frozen Yogurt Bark with Berries (p. 56)
22	Chia Seed Pudding with Almonds and Strawberries (p. 25)	Egg Salad on Whole Grain Crackers (p. 32)	One-Pan Lemon Chicken with Asparagus (p. 40)	Carrot Sticks with Almond Dip (p. 48)	Peanut Butter Banana Bites (p. 56)
23	Whole Grain English Muffin with Peanut Butter and Sliced Banana (p. 25)	Chicken Caesar Salad with Kale (p. 33)	Beef Stir-Fry with Broccoli (p. 41)	Edamame with Sea Salt (p. 48)	Coconut Flour Brownies (p. 57)
24	Sweet Potato and Egg Hash (p. 26)	Sweet Potato and Black Bean Bowl (p. 33)	Vegetarian Chili with Black Beans and Quinoa (p. 41)	Avocado and Cottage Cheese Bowl (p. 49)	Ricotta and Berry Parfait (p. 57)
25	Omelette with Spinach and Feta (p. 26)	Quinoa-Stuffed Bell Peppers (p. 34)	Roasted Chicken Thighs with Brussels Sprouts (p. 42)	Almonds and Dark Chocolate (p. 49)	Almond Joy Energy Bites (p. 58)
26	Protein Pancakes with Almond Flour (p. 27)	Salmon Salad with Avocado and Cucumber (p. 34)	Shrimp and Vegetable Skewers (p. 42)	Tuna Salad Lettuce Cups (p. 50)	Coconut Macaroons (p. 58)

27	Quinoa Breakfast Bowl with Berries and Nuts (p. 27)	Spinach and Feta Stuffed Chicken Breast (p. 35)	Pork Tenderloin with Roasted Carrots (p. 43)	Celery Sticks with Peanut Butter (p. 50)	Frozen Banana Pops with Dark Chocolate (p. 59)
28	Smoked Salmon and Avocado Bagel (p. 28)	Veggie Stir-Fry with Tofu (p. 35)	Chickpea and Spinach Curry (p. 43)	Bell Peppers with Cream Cheese (p. 51)	Pumpkin Spice Energy Balls (p. 59)
29	Low-Carb Egg Muffin Cups (p. 28)	Cauliflower Rice Bowl with Grilled Chicken (p. 36)	Tilapia with Sautéed Kale (p. 44)	Mixed Nuts and Seeds (p. 51)	Berry Coconut Smoothie Bowl (p. 60)
30	Veggie-Packed Egg Muffins (p. 21)	Mushroom and Barley Soup (p. 36)	Turkey and Spinach Stuffed Zucchini Boats (p. 44)	Tomato and Mozzarella Salad (p. 52)	Cinnamon-Spiced Baked Pears (p. 60)

US STANDARD MEASUREMENT CONVERSION

Common Volume Conversions

1 teaspoon (tsp) = 5 milliliters (ml)

1 tablespoon (tbsp) = 3 teaspoons = 15 milliliters (ml)

1 fluid ounce (fl oz) = 2 tablespoons = 30 milliliters (ml)

1/4 cup = 4 tablespoons = 60 milliliters (ml)

1/3 cup = 5 tablespoons + 1 teaspoon = 80 milliliters (ml)

1/2 cup = 8 tablespoons = 120 milliliters (ml)

3/4 cup = 12 tablespoons = 180 milliliters (ml)

1 cup = 16 tablespoons = 240 milliliters (ml)

1 pint = 2 cups = 480 milliliters (ml)

1 quart = 2 pints = 4 cups = 960 milliliters (ml)

1 gallon = 4 quarts = 16 cups = 3.8 liters (l)

Common Weight Conversions

1 ounce (oz) = 28 grams (g)

1 pound (lb) = 16 ounces = 454 grams (g)

Common Length Conversions

1 inch (in) = 2.54 centimeters (cm)

Temperature Conversions

To convert from Fahrenheit to Celsius:

- To convert from Fahrenheit to Celsius: $C = (F - 32) \times \frac{5}{9}$
- To convert from Celsius to Fahrenheit: $F = C \times \frac{9}{5} + 32$

WORKOUT TO MANAGE PREDIABETES

These activities focus on better insulin sensitivity, weight management, and circulatory health, which are key in controlling prediabetes:

Brisk Walking (30-45 minutes, 5 days a week)

Why it works: Walking is a low-impact workout that helps lower blood sugar levels and improve insulin sensitivity. It is simple to begin and may be carried out anyplace.

Action plan: Start with 15-20 minutes of walking daily and gradually increase to 30-45 minutes.

Strength Training (2-3 times per week)

Why it works: Building muscle strength through resistance workouts improves glucose metabolism and helps keep a healthy weight.

Action plan: Incorporate basic movements like squats, lunges, and push-ups, or use resistance bands or light weights.

Bodyweight Squats

Why it works: Squats involve multiple big muscle groups, including the quads, legs, and hips, which help improve glucose metabolism.

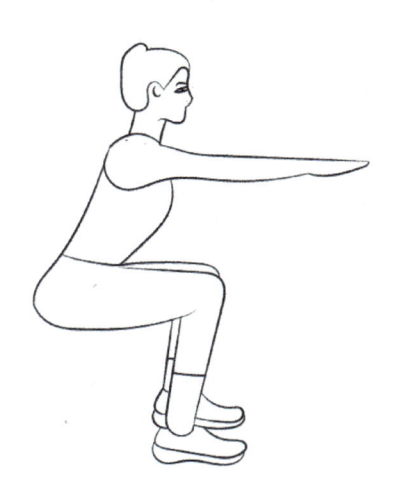

How to do it:

1. Place your feet shoulder-width apart as you stand.
2. Bending your hips and knees as if you were seated can help you lower your body.
3. Once your thighs are parallel to the floor, keep your back straight and descend. To get back up to your feet, push through them.
4. **Reps:** Build up to three sets of fifteen to twenty repetitions, starting with ten to fifteen.

Push-Ups

Why it works: Push-ups improve the chest, shoulders, and arms while working your core, improving total upper-body power and glucose utilization.

How to do it:

1. Start in a plank position with your hands placed shoulder-width apart.
2. Lower your body toward the ground while keeping your back flat, then push yourself back up to the starting position.
3. **Reps:** Start with 8-10 reps, and increase to 2-3 sets of 15-20 reps as you build power.

Lunges

Why it works: Lunges target the legs and hips, helping to improve balance, power, and insulin sensitivity by working large muscle groups.

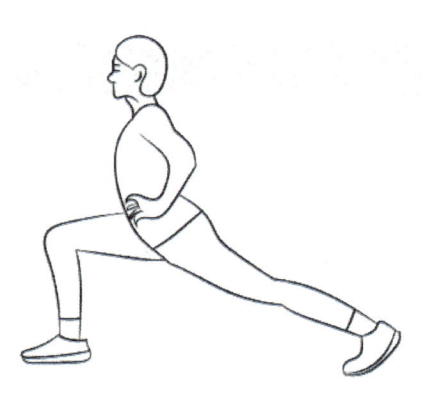

How to do it:

1. Stand up straight and step forward with one leg.
2. Lower your hips until both knees form roughly 90-degree angles.
3. Press through your front heel to return to the starting position, then switch legs.
4. **Reps:** Do 10-12 reps per leg, advancing to 3 sets as you build power.

Dumbbell Rows

Why it works: This exercise targets the back muscles and arms, promoting better balance and upper body power.

How to do it:

1. Hold a dumbbell in each hand, bend slightly forward at the waist, keeping your back straight.
2. Pull the dumbbells toward your waist, keeping your elbows close to your body.
3. Slowly bring them back down.
4. **Reps:** Perform 2-3 sets of 10-12 reps.

Plank

Why it works: Planks build strength in the core, lower back, and shoulders, enhancing stability, balance, and overall strength.

How to do it:

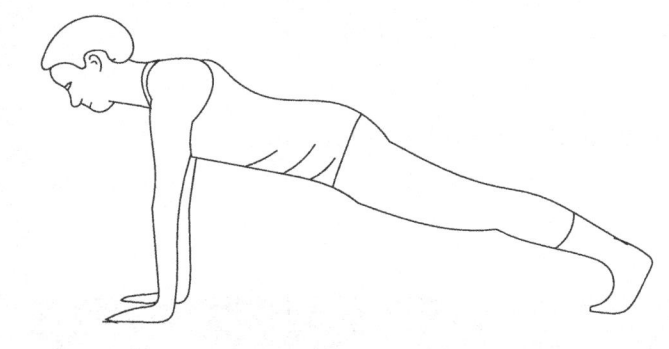

1. Begin in a forearm plank position with your elbows aligned under your shoulders.
2. Maintain a straight line from head to heels, engaging your core.
3. Hold this position for as long as you can.
4. **Reps:** Start with 20-30 seconds, and gradually raise to 1-2 minutes over time.

These routines can be done with minimal tools and can be changed to suit different fitness levels. Incorporating them into your weekly routine 2-3 times per week will help you improve strength and control prediabetes successfully.

YOGA OR PILATES (2 TIMES PER WEEK)

Why it works: These types of exercise improve flexibility, lower stress, and increase insulin sensitivity by increasing muscle use and rest.

Action plan: Try a beginner's yoga or Pilates class or follow guided lessons online. Focus on poses that activate the belly and improve circulation.

Cat-Cow Pose (Yoga)

Why it works: This gentle flow between two poses helps stretch the spine, improve balance, and increase blood flow, which can help in better glucose control.

How to do it:

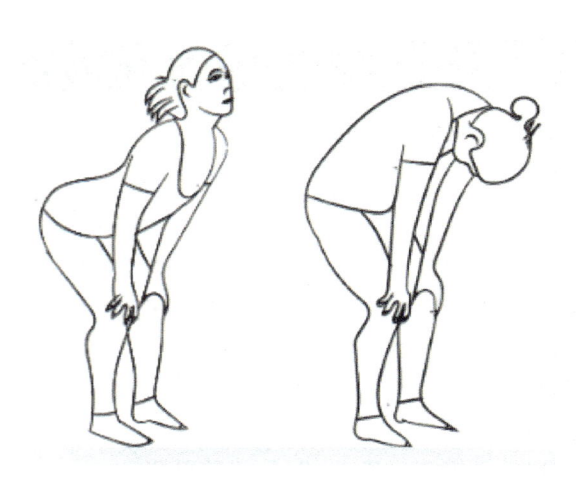

1. Begin in a tabletop position on your hands and knees. Inhale as you arch your back, lifting your head and tailbone (Cow pose).
2. Exhale as you round your spine, tucking your chin to your chest and drawing your belly toward your spine (Cat pose).
3. Repeat this sequence.
4. **Reps:** Perform for 1-2 minutes.

Bridge Pose (Yoga)

Why it works: This pose strengthens the glutes, lower back, and legs, helping improve core stability and insulin sensitivity.

How to do it:

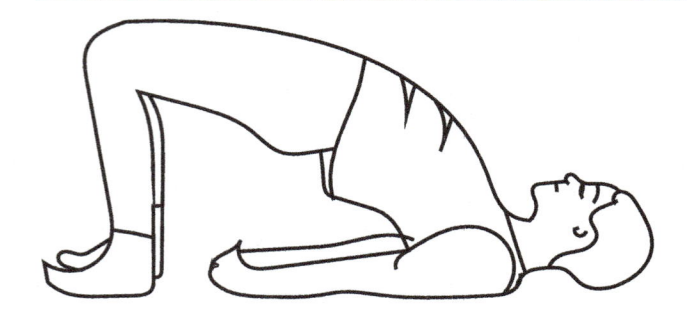

1. Lie on your back with your knees bent and feet flat on the ground, hip-width apart.
2. Press into your feet, lift your hips toward the ceiling, and squeeze your glutes.
3. Hold for a few seconds, then lower back down.
4. **Reps:** Hold for 20-30 seconds, repeated 3-5 times.

The Hundred (Pilates)

Why it works: This Pilates exercise strengthens the core and increases circulation, which can aid in better blood sugar control.

How to do it:

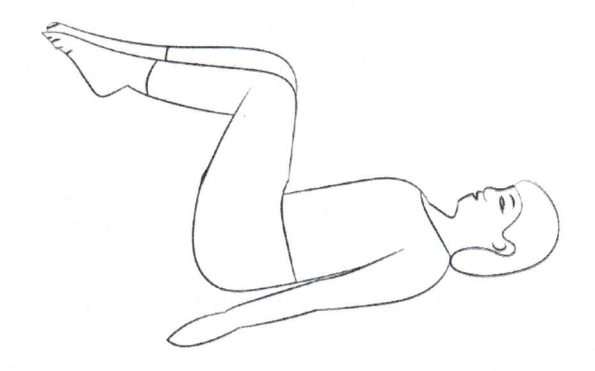

1. Lie on your back with your legs lifted at a 45-degree angle, and arms extended by your sides.
2. Lift your head and shoulders off the mat, and begin moving your arms up and down in small motions while breathing in for 5 counts and out for 5 counts.
3. **Reps:** Continue for 100 pumps (10 full breaths).

Child's Pose (Yoga)

Why it works: A relaxing, healing pose that lowers stress, which is important for controlling blood sugar levels.

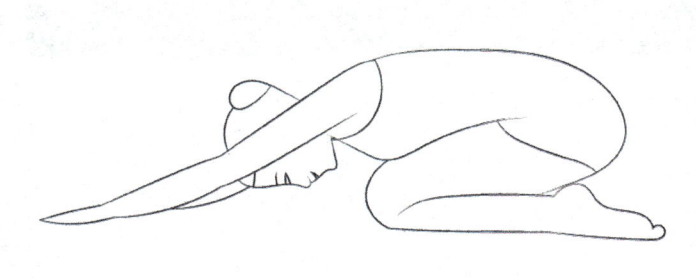

How to do it:

1. Begin in a kneeling position with your big toes touching and knees apart.
2. Sit back onto your heels and reach your arms forward, lowering your forehead to the floor.
3. **Reps:** Hold for 1-3 minutes, focused on deep, calming breaths.

Leg Circles (Pilates)

Why it works: This Pilates move strengthens the core and hips, improving general muscle tone and flexibility, which can support better glucose metabolism.

How to do it:

1. Lie on your back with one leg extended on the ground and the other lifted toward the ceiling.
2. Slowly circle the raised leg in one direction, keeping your core engaged and hips steady.
3. Repeat in the opposite way.
4. **Reps:** Perform 5-10 rounds in each direction for each leg.

Incorporating these movements 2-3 times per week will not only help with flexibility and strength but also lower stress levels, which is crucial in controlling prediabetes.

Cycling (3-4 times per week, 30-60 minutes)

Why it works: Cycling is a great aerobic workout that burns calories, lowers body fat, and improves insulin sensitivity.

Action plan: Start with shorter rides (10-15 minutes) and gradually increase time and effort as stamina improves.

Swimming (2-3 times per week)

Why it works: Swimming offers a full-body workout, burns calories, and is gentle on the joints. It's beneficial for those with joint pain or arthritis.

Action plan: Swim at a gentle pace for 20-30 minutes, gradually increasing time as health improves.

Jump Rope (2-3 times per week, 10-15 minutes)

Why it works: Jump rope is a full-body exercise workout that burns calories quickly and improves heart health.

Action plan: Start with 5-minute sessions and gradually build up to 10-15 minutes, focused on regularity and proper form.

HIIT (HIGH-INTENSITY INTERVAL TRAINING) (2 TIMES PER WEEK)

Why it works: HIIT involves short bursts of hard exercise followed by periods of rest, which can quickly improve insulin sensitivity and promote fat loss.

Action plan: Start with 15–20-minute HIIT workouts, including activities like jumping jacks, runs, or burpees, and rest for similar amounts of time between sets.

Jumping Jacks

Why it works: Jumping jacks raise your heart rate quickly and engage multiple muscle groups, making it a great full-body workout for better insulin sensitivity.

How to do it:

1. Place your feet together and your arms by your sides as you stand.
2. Lift your arms high and leap with your feet out.
3. Return to the beginning location and do it again.
4. **Reps:** Perform for 30 seconds at high effort, followed by 15-30 seconds of rest. Repeat 3-5 times.

Burpees

Why it works: Burpees are a full-body workout that blends cardio and strength, making it effective for raising metabolism and improving glucose control.

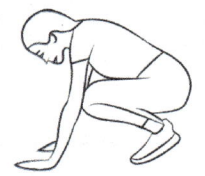

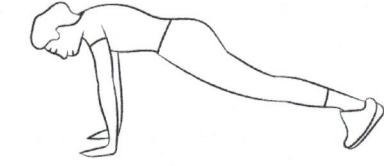

How to do it:

1. Begin by standing, then lower into a squat and place your hands on the floor.
2. Jump your feet back into a plank, do a push-up, then jump your feet back toward your hands and explosively jump into the air.
3. **Reps:** Perform for 30 seconds, rest for 15-30 seconds, and repeat for 3-5 rounds.

High Knees

Why it works: High knees improve physical fitness and increase insulin sensitivity by getting your heart rate up and working core muscles.

How to do it:

1. Stand with your feet hip-width apart.
2. Run in place by lifting your knees toward your chest as high as you can while pumping your arms.
3. **Reps:** Perform for 30 seconds, rest for 15-30 seconds, and repeat for 3-5 rounds.

Mountain Climbers

Why it works: Mountain climbers engage your core, hips, and legs, giving a full-body workout that burns calories and improves insulin sensitivity.

How to do it:

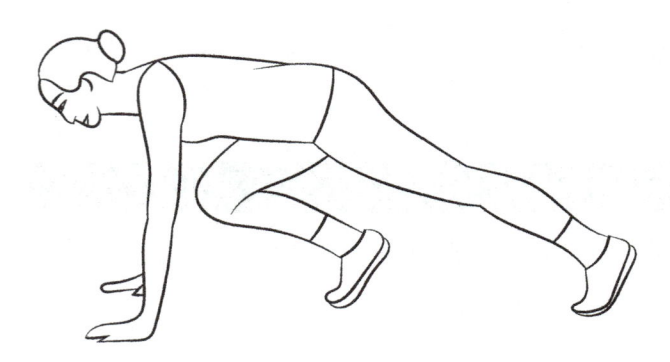

1. Start in a plank position with your arms straight.
2. Pull one knee toward your chest, then quickly switch to the other leg, imitating a running motion.
3. **Reps:** Perform for 30 seconds, rest for 15-30 seconds, and repeat for 3-5 rounds.

Squat Jumps

Why it works: Squat jumps strengthen the legs and hips while raising your heart rate, which can help in controlling blood sugar and promoting fat loss.

How to do it:

1. Place your feet shoulder-width apart as you stand.
2. Drop into a squat, then leap upward with great force, raising your arms over your head.
3. After a gentle landing, immediately begin the next squat.
4. **Reps:** Perform for 30 seconds, rest for 15-30 seconds, and repeat for 3-5 rounds.

These HIIT workouts can be done in a short amount of time but are highly effective for improving aerobic fitness, burning fat, and controlling glucose. Incorporate them into your routine 2-3 times a week for best effects.

Dancing (3-4 times per week, 30 minutes)

Why it works: Dancing is a fun way to burn calories, improve physical health, and boost happiness, lowering the chance of diabetes.

Action plan: Follow online dance classes or join a neighborhood group. Focus on steady moving for 20-30 minutes.

RESISTANCE BAND TRAINING (2-3 TIMES PER WEEK)

Why it works: Resistance band workouts help build lean muscle mass, which improves glucose metabolism and supports insulin sensitivity.

Action plan: Use strength bands to perform workouts like arm curls, leg lifts, and shoulder pushes.

Resistance Band Squats

Why it works: Squats with an elastic band target the hips, quads, and hamstrings, which are big muscle groups that help with glucose metabolism.

How to do it:

1. Place the resistance band under your feet and hold the handles at shoulder height.
2. Perform a squat by lowering your hips back and down, keeping your chest lifted, and then standing back up against the resistance.
3. Reps: Perform 10-12 reps, finishing 2-3 sets.

Resistance Band Rows

Why it works: This practice improves the back muscles and arms, improving balance and general upper body power.

How to do it:

1. Attach the resistance band to a stable anchor (like a door).
2. Stand with feet shoulder-width apart and hold the handles with both hands. Maintaining your elbows close to your body, pull the band toward your chest before going back to the beginning position.
3. Reps: Perform 10-12 reps, finishing 2-3 sets.

Resistance Band Chest Press

Why it works: Chest presses target the chest, shoulders, and arms, helping to build upper body power and improve insulin sensitivity.

How to do it:

1. Anchor the pressure band behind you at chest height.
2. Hold the bars and step forward with one foot for balance.
3. Push the handles forward until your arms are fully stretched, then slowly return to the starting position.
4. Reps: Perform 10-12 reps, finishing 2-3 sets.

Resistance Band Lateral Walks

Why it works: This practice improves the glutes and hip muscles, helping with flexibility and lower body power.

How to do it:

1. Place a resistance band around your legs just above your knees.
2. Place your feet shoulder-width apart and slant your knees slightly. Step to the side, keeping tension in the band, and then step the other foot to meet the first.
3. Repeat in the opposite way.
4. Reps: Perform 10-15 steps in each direction, finishing 2-3 times.

Resistance Band Bicep Curls

Why it works: This workout targets the arms, helping to improve upper body power and muscle tone.

How to do it:

1. Stand on the resistance band with feet shoulder-width apart and hold the handles with your hands facing upward.
2. Curl the handles toward your shoulders, keeping your arms close to your sides, and then slowly lower the handles back down.
3. Reps: Perform 10-12 reps, finishing 2-3 sets.

These resistance band workouts are low-impact and easy to change for different fitness levels, making them ideal for those controlling prediabetes.

CONCLUSION:

You're now on a path to not only fix prediabetes but also live a better, more satisfying life. By now, you should have a better idea of how your food, exercise routine, and daily habits can help your health and blood sugar levels. Every small change you make, like changing your meals to meet special food needs, working exercise into your busy schedule, or learning how to deal with stress, brings you closer to long-term health.

Inspiration to Make Healthy Choices for Life

The main thing you should remember from this guide is that growth is a process, not a goal. Managing prediabetes and lowering the chance of getting type 2 diabetes both depend on making changes to your lifestyle so that you can keep up. It's important to keep your eye on the big picture, even if there are problems along the way. You can build a better life with every healthy choice you make, like choosing whole foods, getting more exercise, or finding ways to relax and deal with stress.

Celebrate small wins: Don't overlook the power of small successes. Even the smallest change in your food, exercise, or stress control counts as growth. It takes time for these small changes to add up to big changes.

Stay consistent: What makes you successful is being consistent, not being perfect. If you slip up or face a failure, don't focus on it—just get back on track with the next meal or exercise session.

Stay flexible: Life is uncertain, and keeping flexibility in your approach to health can help you stay on course. Allow yourself to adapt to new conditions without guilt or anger.

Remember, it's not about hardship or strict diets but about building a healthy, fun lifestyle that supports your health goals. As you continue this journey, keep looking for ways to improve and support your health.

FINAL THOUGHTS AND WORDS OF WISDOM FROM ANTONETTE BATZ

I've had the honor of assisting several individuals in changing their lives by addressing their diet and lifestyle choices as a certified nutritionist and diabetes care specialist. I want to inform you that you can alter the outcomes of your health. Prediabetes doesn't define you, and it certainly isn't a permanent disease. With the right attitude, determination, and tactics, you can take control of your health and avoid the development of type 2 diabetes.

Here are a few basic ideas I'd like you to take with you:

Focus on Nourishment, Not Restriction: Instead of thinking about what you can't eat, focus on all the wonderful, healthy foods that fuel your body. Whole grains, lean meats, healthy fats, and fresh vegetables can change your meals and keep you refreshed.

Prioritize Self-Care: Taking care of your mental, social, and physical well-being is important in controlling prediabetes. Remember, worry and lack of sleep can affect blood sugar as much as food and exercise. Build habits that promote self-care and mental health.

Find Joy in the Process: Cooking healthy meals, staying busy, and caring for yourself should be fun. Find the joy in finding new foods, trying new forms of movement, and taking care of your body.

Build a Support System: Don't go through this process alone. Surround yourself with a community of family, friends, or even online groups who support you and hold you responsible.

Be Patient with Yourself: Sustainable change takes time. Trust the process, be patient, and remember that mistakes are part of the trip.

Your health is in your hands, and I'm sure that by following the principles described in this guide, you will create a life that is not only better but also more energetic and fun."

Your road to health starts now. With the tools and insights, you've gained, you're prepared to make lasting changes that can fix prediabetes and improve your general well-being. Take each day as a chance to invest in your health, and remember that every healthy choice you make is a step toward a brighter, better future.

Made in United States
North Haven, CT
07 May 2025

68642406R00057